Interpreting the Medical Literature

Interpreting the Medical Literature

FIFTH EDITION

Stephen H. Gehlbach, MD, MPH
University of Massachusetts
Amherst, Massachusetts

McGraw-Hill
Medical Publishing Division

*New York Chicago San Francisco Lisbon London Madrid
Mexico City Milan New Delhi San Juan Seoul
Singapore Sydney Toronto*

Interpreting the Medical Literature, Fifth Edition

Copyright © 2006 by The McGraw-Hill Companies, Inc. All rights reserved. Printed in the United States of America. Except as permitted under the United States Copyright Act of 1976, no part of this publication may be reproduced or distributed in any form or by any means, or stored in a database or retrieval system, without the prior written permission of the publisher.

1 2 3 4 5 6 7 8 9 0   DOC/DOC   0 9 8 7 6

ISBN: 0-07-143789-4

This book was set in Times Roman by International Typesetting and Composition.
The editors were James F. Shanahan and Peter J. Boyle.
The production supervisor was Catherine Saggese.
Project management was provided by International Typesetting and Composition.
The index was prepared by Susan Hunter.
RR Donnelley was printer and binder.
This book is printed on acid-free paper.

Library of Congress Cataloging-in-Publication Data

Gehlbach, Stephen H.
  Interpreting the medical literature / Stephen H. Gehlbach.—5th ed.
    p. ; cm.
  Includes bibliographical references and index.
  ISBN 0-07-143789-4 (pbk.)
  1. Medical literature. 2. Medicine—Research. 3. Epidemiology—Terminology. I. Title.
  [DNLM: 1. Research Design. 2. Meta-Analysis. 3. Publications. W 20.5 G31li 2006]
  R118.6.G43 2006
  610.72—dc22

                                                                    2005056121

Contents

CHAPTER NINE
Analysis: Some Statistical Tests **161**

CHAPTER TEN
Interpretation: Sensitivity, Specificity, and Predictive Value **177**

CHAPTER ELEVEN
Interpretation: Risk **203**

CHAPTER TWELVE
Interpretation: Causes **225**

Preface

It has been almost a quarter of a century since this book first came out and though things have changed they also have remained the same. Medical research and the reports it generates have grown in volume and complexity. There is much more to read. Designs are more rigorous. Statistical analyses have become considerably more sophisticated. This is good news; it means that the quality of much of the research has improved. Yet the need remains as strong as ever to cultivate the critical skills to read and interpret this literature. No matter how elaborate the trappings, the value of an article still depends on fundamentals of good design—on proper selection and organization of subjects, on the quality of data collection, and on the valid interpretation of results. These principles have not changed; they remain firmly at the center of intelligent reading.

The book remains a basic epidemiology text at heart. I have resisted temptations to make it more complex, forgoing detailed explorations into areas such as meta-analysis, cost-effectiveness analysis, decision analysis, and statistical modeling. These topics are introduced, but the emphasis remains on the fundamentals.

Originally, the book was written for a specific audience—medical students and practicing clinicians. With increasing discussions of "critical appraisal" and "evidence-based medicine" in clinical circles, these readers should continue to find it useful. Happily, other groups have also found the book valuable. Public health students, nurses, pharmacists, workers in the pharmaceutical industry, and even attorneys have gained assistance in negotiating the maze of medical research.

In this last quarter-century the Internet has clearly transformed access to medical research. Much of the information found only by hours of prowling in library stacks 25 years ago is now available at an instant from one's desk. The Internet has been of great assistance in compiling this new edition. The National Library of Medicine with its PubMed site, as well as online resources of a number of medical journals, have been invaluable. But I have not attempted to catalog, evaluate, or incorporate into the text the many streams of electronic information that rush at lay and professional audiences. The currents are too rapid and too changeable. The accompanying caveat is that, while the Internet gives us access to information with unprecedented ease, validity is not assured. Critical appraisal is still required. If anything, the need grows more pressing as the cascade grows.

The book relies on published medical and public health literature for most of its examples. I believe that these are more compelling than artificial illustrations and have included only a few concocted examples—as much to lighten the tone as to illuminate. The challenge continues to keep the examples up-to-date. Choices to retain or discard those that have "seen some use" are difficult. Some articles, despite their age, relate to topics that are of continuing interest. Others illustrate principles and points so well that they are difficult to displace. Still others are such classics I cannot bear to part with them. However, some articles of diminished luster have been replaced with more recent illustrations.

Another caveat: Because this book uses published studies to teach critical appraisal, it occasionally might appear uncomplimentary toward the efforts of colleagues. No use of illustrations in the book should be taken as disparaging. Conducting research is a formidable task. The difficulties inherent in studying and documenting the behavior of humans are legion and the achievement of perfection, rare. Few studies are beyond comment. It is important that as we hone our critical skills, we develop equipoise— a sense of the balance between the strengths and limitations of any study. Despite what sometimes seems a daunting list of potential liabilities, most articles have value. Our task is to discover it. Some goodwill is necessary; this and the application of the appraisal skills the book provides should net productive reading of the medical literature.

CHAPTER ONE

Tasting an Article

*Some books are to be tasted, others to be swallowed, and some
few to be chewed and digested.*

FRANCIS BACON

Keeping up with the medical literature is a strenuous proposition. The stacks of unread journals that collect on desks and in filing cabinets only grow larger. The number of textbooks, yearbooks, newsletters, and specialty journals swells, while the time to read them shrinks. The explosion of information available on the Internet adds exponentially to the burden. Yet we are pressed to keep current from many sides. Most of us are taught early in our education that to be a competent professional, one must keep abreast of the latest in clinical syndromes, causal theories, novel diagnostic tests, innovative treatments, and risks of adverse events. We need to learn which environmental carcinogens to avoid and how to improve our understanding of the causes of heart disease. Specialty examinations and licensure requirements reinforce this concept. Some recertification plans specifically call for examinations based on information from the current literature.

Patients expect physicians to be informed. Like their doctors, patients are beset with medical facts and fiction from radio, television, the popular press, and the World Wide Web. Whether they read the *New York Times* or a supermarket tabloid, they are likely to be getting information that is at least in part based on reports from the medical literature. Patients want to know about the risk of contracting Lyme disease when they visit Connecticut, whether their headaches deserve an MRI examination, or whether there are serious side effects from the medicine they've just been prescribed.

Even though the spirit may be willing, the eyes grow weak, and the task of sorting through the mounds of published material seems a losing affair. Some remedy would appear to come from the many secondary sources that are available. Medical textbooks, review journals, newsletters, audiocassettes, and Web sites supply synthesized information on current topics. One can easily read the collected opinions of experts about everything from ankylosing spondylitis to tropical zoonoses from one of several excellent texts, or by listening to a learned colleague while driving to work, thanks to the wonders of magnetic tape. The views of gurus gathered together by the National Institutes of Health as a consensus panel to pronounce on the proper diagnosis and treatment of osteoporosis are available on a U.S. government Web site. Secondary sources are an efficient way to gather information and circumvent the painful process of trying to master the presentation of data in primary sources. Experts have problems like the rest of us. Sometimes their subjective selves get the upper hand and cast controversy into fact. Opinions and biased reading can become standard knowledge. That should not surprise us. Studies on the same subject may present conflicting findings or be open to differing interpretations. It does mean, however, that while texts, reviews, and expert panels are useful, we cannot depend entirely on secondary sources for our information. We need to be able to evaluate a primary research article ourselves and judge its value.

Finding time to do this reading is not the only challenge. Articles describing research studies have become increasingly sophisticated. Not only has the complexity of the information presented increased, but the methods used to obtain and interpret data have also become correspondingly complex. Studies now utilize "stratified sampling techniques," "randomized double-blind crossover designs," and a multitude of semicomprehensible techniques for statistical analysis. Understanding the nuances of these methodologies is every bit as demanding as keeping up with the side effects of the latest pharmacological agents or the newest discoveries of immune-cell function.

The purpose of this book is to give practical aid to the beleaguered seeker of medical knowledge. This chapter offers advice on general approaches to reading articles—on exercising our powers of selectivity and efficiency.

As Francis Bacon suggested some 400 years ago, much of the written material that comes our way deserves only a perfunctory taste, with relatively few articles meriting full digestion.

Once we have developed some rules for making initial decisions about which articles to read and have gained an overall sense of what they are about, we can proceed with a more detailed critical review. The chapters that follow will be devoted to exploring the design of studies, classifying methodologies, and learning about their basic strengths and weaknesses. Ways in which data are analyzed and interpreted will be major areas of emphasis. Issues such as statistical significance, risk, causation, and predictive value will be discussed.

The goal of all this will be to arrive at an interpretation we can call our own. We will balance the strengths and flaws uncovered in an article and come up with an independent assessment of whether the author's message rings true—whether in the final analysis acupuncture successfully reduces pain or treating mild hypertension lowers morbidity from stroke. The bottom line is validity. Are the results believable? Do they represent the truth? Are they applicable to our practice? Will the patients we see and treat respond in the same way as those described in the study? Does the paper really support its claims?

REASONS TO READ

We have addressed the general goal of keeping current as a reason for reading journals. Medical journals offer more than reports of recent information on tests, treatments, and concepts of etiology. They provide a fascinating potpourri of opinion, philosophy, argument, gossip, history, theory, and advice. We have mentioned the topical review articles that condense up-to-date thoughts on the treatment of congestive heart failure or use of ultrasound technology. Practical hints, such as diagnosing scabies in the office or setting up pension plans for employees, are features of some journals. Comments published as letters to the journal and sage remarks made by the editors can make engaging and informative reading. These are especially valuable when they offer informed critiques of research articles or when authors debate the results of research in an open forum. There are pieces that discuss aspects of the history of the profession, such as a review of smallpox immunization in early Boston, views from other parts of the medical world, or philosophical pieces on the wonders and frailties of our medical system.

That is a splendid array of offerings, and we have not mentioned the book reviews, employment opportunities, and news of professional organizations. Any part of this list makes legitimate reading, but none falls into the category of primary research, which is the meat of our discussion. Among the new ideas and information available to readers are the choices listed in Table 1-1. They span a spectrum—from learning about Avian influenza and African tick-bite fever to sharing facts about physician-assisted suicides. .

This rich smorgasbord is worth noting, since reasons for picking up a journal will vary. The approach one takes to reading an article depends

---

TABLE 1–1

Some reasons for reading medical articles

Read to find out about	For example
New health problems	Avian influenza African tick-bite fever
New presentation or manifestations of diseases	Transfusion-transmitted malaria Childhood viruses in adults
Extent and natural history of health problems	Prevalence of HIV among university students Cognitive function after coronary artery bypass surgery
Tests for diagnosis and prognosis	Screening for alcohol abuse Ruling out myocardial infarction
New treatments or programs	St. John's wort for depression Statins for aortic stenosis
Adverse effects of medical care	Safety of "COX2" inhibitors Hospital characteristics and adverse events
Causes (and noncauses) and predictors of disease	Cancer risk from passive smoking Heart failure from emotional distress
Experience of others	Ultrasound in recurrent abdominal pain Physician-assisted suicide
Expert recommendations	Adjuvant therapy for breast cancer Managing insomnia

very much on the intent at the outset. Reading to review the pathophysiology of Epstein-Barr virus infection or to learn what an expert committee views as the proper approach to identifying and treating high levels of cholesterol in the blood is a different process from assessing the validity of a report linking infant feeding practices to later childhood obesity. Deciding in advance what you wish to obtain from the journal is the first step to more efficient reading.

Understanding the framework of articles also facilitates efficiency. Mortimer J. Adler has produced an entire volume on how to read a book.[1] In it, he emphasizes that effective reading requires identifying and understanding the structure or components of a work. That, he states, contributes to the "intelligibility of the whole." Adler's advice on reading books has parallels for the reader of medical journals. His medical metaphor to approaching a great book has an irresistible message:

> Every book has a skeleton hidden between its boards. Your job is to find it. A book comes to you with flesh on its bare bones and clothes over its flesh. It is all dressed up. I am not asking you to be impolite or cruel. You do not have to undress it or tear the flesh off its limbs to get at the firm structure that underlies the soft. But you must read the book with x-ray eyes, for it is an essential part of your first apprehension of any book to grasp its structure.[1]

THE BONES OF AN ARTICLE

Most articles that deliver new information to readers share a basic structural plan. The six main sections outlined in Table 1-2 are usually present.

The *summary* or *abstract* should present a concise statement of the goal or hypothesis of the study, a word or two about how the endeavor was undertaken, highlights of the results, and a concluding thought that puts it all into perspective. To facilitate this, many journals have introduced "structured abstracts." While the formats for these vary from journal to journal, they generally organize information by useful headings such as "Study Objective," "Design," and "Results." Not only do structured abstracts provide readers with a useful guide but they also encourage authors to attend to details about method that are sometimes overlooked. Readers should be able to glean a reasonable sense of the contents of a journal by

TABLE 1–2	
The basic structure of an article	
Section	**Look for the following**
Abstract/Summary	Overview or summary of the work Highlights of results General statement of significance
Introduction	Background information: history, pathophysiology, clinical presentation Review of the work of others Rationale for present study
Methods/Materials & Methods/ Patients & Methods	Study design Subject selection procedures Methods of measurement Description of analytic techniques
Results	What happened? Graphics—tables, charts, figures—that sum- marize findings
Discussion/Comment/Conclusion	Meaning, significance of work Critique of study: discussion of limitations as well as strengths, further analysis Comparison with work of others Disclaimers, equivocation, apologies, chest thumping, speculation, instruction, fantasy, and so on
References/Bibliography	Evidence that work of others has been considered Lead to further exploration of the subject

flipping past the antacid advertisements and scanning just the abstracts. One could do worse than be a nibbler of abstracts. One sometimes needs to do better, however. Abstracts provide a useful taste of the contents of the study, but they are rarely sufficient to make a meal in themselves. Because of the need to be concise, abstracts select only the highlights of a paper. They are also, quite understandably, an author's attempt to put his best foot forward.

Sometimes the summary of the article contains more wish than reality and presents a distorted view of the work that follows. Evidence of this problem was uncovered when abstracts from six widely read medical journals were evaluated.[2] Investigators looked for data discrepancies between the body of the article and the abstract. They found that deficiencies were unhappily common, ranging from 18 to 68% (typically 30–40%). Types of sins uncovered were principally those where data either were inconsistent between the two sources or where data presented in the abstract were not found in the body of the work at all. Deception is probably not intended, but vigorous condensation sometimes imparts a false flavor.

The *introduction* section of the paper usually provides background information on the topic to be addressed, as well as rationale for why the authors undertook the adventure. Sometimes the introduction will offer an extended review of other literature surrounding the topic. When well done, this provides readers with a nourishing appetizer before they undertake the main course of the paper; it may, in itself, make the reading worthwhile.

The next section describes the *methodology* of the study. It is labeled "Materials and Methods," "Patients and Methods," or some other variation on that theme. It details the patient populations studied, study designs utilized, and data collection techniques employed; it describes in more detail than many of us care to know the analytical and evaluative procedures used in the course of the study. This is the section that many readers skip. In fact, it is the section that some journals relegate to small print. It is also the section to which we will devote much of our analytical energy and to which we will return repeatedly in future chapters.

The *results* section, quite logically, presents the information obtained from the execution of the study. Results are usually found both in the text and in accompanying tables, charts, graphs, and figures. Analysis and some interpretation of the data are also presented in this section. Like the methods section, this section represents an essential part of the main bill of fare and will be discussed at considerable length.

An interesting mix of ingredients can go into fashioning the *discussion* or *comment* section of an article. A further analysis of the results may be accomplished; results and conclusions of other studies may be compared and contrasted; the authors may offer apologies for oversights and transgressions or build a case to strengthen and support results. The discussion section is usually the most speculative and often the most interesting reading in the medical paper. Authors may review and comment upon other studies related to their own work and try to place the results in perspective. It can make especially entertaining reading if the authors' interpretation of the work is quite different from your own.

A list of *references* or a *bibliography* usually finishes off an article. Little more need be said about the references except that they are most conspicuous by their absence. Few authors are writing on topics so novel that some thought and other research has not gone on before. The list of references gives a reader a clue to how diligently authors have researched and reviewed the experience of other workers. An extensive, well-done bibliography that provides easy access to a wide selection of articles on a topic can save hunting through library reference works and is sometimes the saving grace of an otherwise lackluster journal article. When articles are accessed from the Internet, direct links from references to abstracts and articles can provide an irresistible sojourn into related work.

Having a firm idea of what you wish to gain from reading a journal and knowing how to utilize the framework of an article to best advantage gets you off to a proper start. With this background, a few rules for sampling the literature are needed.

APPROACHING AN ARTICLE

Read Only What Is Interesting and Useful

Whether the cause is overzealous toilet training or an oppressive system of early education, most of us have acquired a disquieting degree of compulsive behavior by the time we reach graduate school or professional practice. This trait is not without value. It helps us master the many facts required to pass our comprehensive examinations, produce a dissertation, or persist in attacking a patient's ketoacidosis at 2 o'clock in the morning. However, compulsiveness has its liabilities as well. Confronted with a burgeoning pile of journals, we cannot bear the thought that any of the information packed within those glossy pages should go unabsorbed. We wait for that magical time when we can sit down and plow through it. That day never arrives, and our guilt grows proportionally with the stack, diminishing only occasionally when a few spare hours enable us to prune the pile by one or two or when a housekeeping purge assigns it all irrevocably to the attic or trash bin. Mental health demands that we become more selective readers. Rather than trying to devour every last article, we need to develop tactics for sampling journals and consuming only those articles that are most nutritious.

Your first taste of an article should have a selective purpose. What is the article about? Is it a topic of interest? Is the information likely to be useful? If an article is not of interest, do not read it! There is plenty of information overloading our synapses as it is. There is no point in burdening the system with information that will not be used. It takes up time and space and probably will not be retained. Of course there is a risk in making choices. The case report dismissed as unworthy after a quick look may well be just like the case of a patient who strolls into your office next Friday or becomes the topic of a discussion at grand rounds. So be it. Selective reading is an even greater problem for students, who must read omnivorously to define their areas of interest and for whom examinations and interrogating professors are ever-present incentives to devour information. The solution to the problem is simple in concept but requires willpower to execute.

1. Scan the table of contents and decide what each article is about.

2. Select articles to be pursued in greater detail and bypass those that are not of interest. (The faint of heart who are reluctant to make this decision on the basis of a title alone may consult the abstract.)

3. Do not equivocate. Do not accumulate a pile of maybes. Articles that might be useful in the future but are of little interest now usually do not get read. All of us like to hedge our bets against that time when we will encounter that rare new genetic syndrome or want to know how to treat a patient with schistosomiasis. Resist temptation. Medical libraries are full of just such advice, and now much of their contents is accessible almost instantaneously from your desktop computer. Pursue such information when the special need arises.

Scan the Article to Gain a Quick Overview

An important corollary to selective reading is to hold back the initial impulse to bite right into an article. Step back for a brief, circumspect view of the whole. You may be surprised at what you discover. Finding page after page of uninterrupted, double-column print may permanently dampen your enthusiasm or relegate the piece to a day when you really do have more time to spend. A quick flip through may tell you that the technical complexity of the article is more than you are prepared to take on. Unintelligible jargon or complicated mathematical formulas may suggest that your reading time would be more profitably spent elsewhere.

You may discover on this quick perusal that an article you thought would offer practical clinical tidbits is actually a report of highly specialized laboratory work. A piece listed in the contents as "Cow's Milk Allergy" turns out to report on "the production of a lymphokine, the leukocyte-migration inhibition factor, by peripheral blood lymphocytes in response to an in vitro challenge with bovine beta-lactoglobulin."[3] Or, an article from which you anticipated exciting new information is only a revival of some well-worn old facts. Look over the graphs and tables. These are particularly useful in giving a perspective, since they are usually carefully selected by authors to summarize the main messages of the piece (worth more than many thousand words, as they say).

Scanning gives the reader a sense of the structure of an article, a perspective in which to organize thoughts. Many articles will, within the basic framework already described, offer subheadings that facilitate this structuring process. Scan them. A competent author, as Adler suggests, has organized the architecture of a work to be a functional, intelligible guide to the whole.

Concentrate on the Methods Section

Once you decide that an article is worth reading—assuming your appetite has not been dulled by the quick scan—a new approach is needed. Most readers begin and end with the abstract. Those with the fortitude to take on more of the article generally proceed to the introduction, then pale at the prospect of reading the small print in the methods section and skip it. Sometimes they also pass over tedious presentations of results in favor of finding, in the spirit of a suspense novel, what happens at the end. Since the author usually rehashes the results and offers an overall interpretation of the study in the discussion section, heading straight for the last section seems an economical way to proceed.

Unfortunately, there is support for this pessimism. A survey that queried over 400 internists practicing in the United States about their journal reading habits revealed that only the abstract was read for 63% of articles.[4] Fitzgerald has supplied evidence that "methods" are often not favored fare.[5] During ward rounds, she passed out an article on diabetic retinopathy to a group of 11 medical students and interns. They were instructed to read the paper and 2 companion articles carefully for discussion at subsequent rounds. As a test of critical reading savvy, Fitzgerald substituted for the methods section of the paper a comparable section from an entirely different article. Only 1 of the 8 learners who read the paper noticed the substitution.

One purpose of this book is to retrain readers to focus on the design and analysis of studies. Read the methods section first. Here is the substance of the research. Any new information, no matter how enthusiastically discussed or fervently endorsed, is only as useful as the study's planning and execution are sound. The design or analysis of an article may be so lacking that no amount of explanation, extrapolation, or apology on the part of the authors can set it right. Our time is better spent elsewhere.

Reserve the Right of Final Judgment

One last and very important principle remains. The ultimate interpretation and decision about the value of an article rests with the reader. Too frequently, we are cowed by the power of the printed word. After all, the author has reviewed the literature, designed and executed the study, and presented a convincing array of results. Who are we to quibble with the interpretation? It is only reasonable to defer to the experts. That is why reading only the introduction and discussion sections of the paper seems so efficient—a little background followed by an erudite discussion of the results.

Do not be fooled! We have every right to pin our own interpretation on the results. The burden of proof is upon the authors to convince us that they are right. The goal of learning to read critically is to develop skills to analyze an article and make an independent assessment of its worthiness. It is a matter of educating the palate.

But a word of caution! It's easy to become overly critical. Finding flaws in a research article is often easier than giving unqualified praise. If we look hard and long enough, we are bound to find some blemishes in the best of reported studies. The challenge is a balanced assessment. As readers, we must acknowledge human imperfection and decide whether, given the limitations of almost any study, the net is valid and useful. In the final analysis, can we believe the results? Is the work applicable to our setting and the kinds of patients we see?

Bear in mind through the next chapters that, although the pitfalls associated with designing, analyzing, and interpreting medical studies seem numerous and the apparent defects in published works many, there is much valuable information for us to chew on and digest.

REFERENCES

1. Adler MJ: *How to Read a Book: The Art of Getting a Liberal Education.* Simon & Schuster, 1940.
2. Pitkin RM, Branagan MA, Burmeister LF: Accuracy of data in abstracts of published research articles. JAMA 1999;281(12):1110.
3. Ashkenazi A et al: In vitro cell-mediated immunologic assay for cow's milk allergy. Pediatrics 1980;65:399.
4. Saint S et al: Journal reading habits of internists. J Gen Intern Med 2000;15(12):881.
5. Fitzgerald FT: From Galen to Xerox: The authoritarian reference in medicine. Ann Intern Med 1982;96:245.

CHAPTER TWO

Study Design: General Considerations

I'll no more on't: it hath made me mad.

HAMLET, ACT III, SCENE I

Although Hamlet may not have been specifically discussing his feelings on the taxonomy of study designs, he could well have been. Sorting through the maze of terms that are commonly employed to describe the design of studies could totter the most stable mind or flutter the stoutest heart. We are likely to encounter references to retrospective and prospective studies, prevalence, case-control and cohort studies, follow-up, and cross-sectional and ecologic studies. Along with longitudinal and incidence studies, there are experimental studies and clinical trials. We even get combinations such as retrospective cohort studies. The list goes on, but at this point most readers are ready to throw their hands skyward in irrevocable despair. How did we arrive at such a confusing state of affairs, and what can a relatively reasonable soul expect to gain from making some sense of the taxonomy of study design?

Epidemiologists are probably most to blame for the glut of terminology. As methodologists they are rightfully concerned with precise definitions of the tools of their trade. And, to be fair, the challenges inherent in studying the complexities of health in human populations are considerable.

Unfortunately, no one in the union seems able to accept the definitions of other members, and the neologisms have sprouted. One article in an epidemiology journal describes and discusses 23 definitions of the word "epidemiology."[1] As is the case with new cars and remedies for colds, the proliferation of terms describing study designs suggests that none is entirely satisfactory.

Although it is tempting to leave this semantic tangle to those who enjoy it, there are several principles about study design that the intelligent reader needs to master. The trick is to keep the forest in view without floundering in the foliage. Identifying the structure of a study gives the reader the jump on assessing the validity of an article. Just as facts about the make and model of an automobile suggest predictive features about its gas mileage, repair record, and comfort, the facts about a study provide insight about strengths to be anticipated and weaknesses to probe for.

Let us begin with an overview to put the elements of study design into perspective. For purposes of discussion we will not haggle about terminology. The goal is to get at the concepts that underlie designs. Table 2–1 supplies a schematic of the basic designs into which most medical studies fall. Many reports in the literature can be designated as descriptive, as seen on the left-hand side of the table.

DESCRIPTIVE STUDIES

As the term suggests, *descriptive* articles serve chiefly to record events, observations, and activities. They do not provide detailed explanations of the causes of disease or offer the kind of evidence we need to evaluate the efficacy of new treatments. They are, however, invaluable documentaries that, once filed, may lead to exciting discoveries. At its least complicated, a *descriptive study* is a report of a case or a small series of cases that an observer feels should be brought to the attention of colleagues. Accounts of an unusual episode of poisoning or an atypical rash developing after administration of a new medication are examples of descriptive studies at their simplest. These reports alert us about possible drug side effects, unusual complications of illnesses, or surprising presentations of diseases. Caution must always be exercised in interpreting a single report or series of cases, since it is not always clear, for example, that the unusual rash or ringing in the ears reported by the patient who has been given a

TABLE 2–1
Basic study designs

EXPLANATORY

Examine etiology, cause, efficacy, using the strategy of comparisons

EXPERIMENTAL

Evaluate efficacy of therapeutic, educational, administrative interventions

Investigator controls allocation

Examples:

Clinical trial
- Efficacy of statins for aortic stenosis
- Surgical vs. medical management of angina

Educational intervention
- Self-instruction vs. lecture on anemia

Healthcare trial
- Nurse practitioner vs. physician care

OBSERVATIONAL

Seek causes, etiologies, predictors, better diagnosis

Investigator observes nature

Examples:

Case-control
- Dietary fiber and colon cancer

Follow-up
- Estrogen use and development of osteoporosis

Cross-sectional
- Astroviruses as a cause of diarrhea

DESCRIPTIVE

Document and communicate experience: share ideas, programs, treatments, unusual events, and observations

Begin search for explanations

Examples:

Case report or series
- Rash developing during drug treatment
- Cluster of cases of Kaposi's sarcoma

Clinical series
- 59 patients with West Nile virus infection

Population
- Prevalence of HIV in military recruits
- Community survey of needs of elderly

Program or course
- Course on sexuality for medical students

new antibiotic is related to the drug. However, the observations first noted in descriptive studies often lead to further, confirmatory work that produces important findings.

Case reports have been around for a long time. Consider William Heberden's account of chest pain occurring in "nearly a hundred people" in the year 1772:[2]

> There is a disorder of the breast marked with strong and peculiar symptoms, considerable for the kind of danger belonging to it, and not extremely rare. . . . They who are afflicted with it, are seized while they are walking (more especially if it be up hill, and soon after eating) with a painful and most disagreeable sensation in the breast which seems as if it would extinguish life, if it were to increase or to continue; but the moment they stand still, all this uneasiness vanishes. . . . In some inveterate cases it has been brought on by the motion of a horse, or a carriage, and even by swallowing, coughing, going to stool, or speaking, or any disturbance of mind.

This elegant description turns out to be the first delineation of the syndrome of angina pectoris.

More recently, a group of physicians noticed an unusual cluster of patients with a rare skin tumor.[3] Not only was the frequency of these cases unexpected, but the course of the disease was atypical. Where the malignancy usually occurs as a slowly growing affliction of men in their sixties or seventies, it suddenly presented as an aggressive, life-threatening disease among homosexual men in their twenties and thirties. This description of 8 cases of Kaposi's sarcoma first alerted the world to a problem of considerable importance.

Another type of descriptive study is the clinical series in which, for example, authors describe the presentation and response to antibiotics of a group of tick-bitten South African travelers who have fever and skin lesions, or the outcome of 100 patients undergoing a new technique for dispensing with gallstones. This is not fancy research, but it creates useful catalogs of the experience of others.

Large populations can also be the subject of descriptive studies. The practicing physicians of Oregon may be questioned regarding their attitudes toward the state's new "death with dignity act." Diagnostic information collected from multiple primary care practices detailing the number of patients with hypertension, diabetes, and acute sore throat may form the basis for "defining content of family practice." Such information may help in making practice-management decisions, such as the need for a dietitian to counsel diabetic patients or how to plan a curriculum for training residents. A description of a new course in human sexuality that has been successfully taught to medical students or a community survey conducted to assess the health needs of the geriatric population are other examples of this type of design. So, in addition to being starting points for more elaborate assaults on the etiology of disease, descriptive studies can be used for a variety of educational, administrative, and health-planning purposes.

EXPLANATORY STUDIES

Comparison is the basic strategy of explanatory studies. These studies seek answers to questions such as which treatment for breast cancer is most effective? Is there a relationship between physical activity and heart disease? What are the factors that predict which patients will miss appointments? Explanatory studies attempt to provide insight into etiology or find better treatments. The methods employed can be grouped into two major approaches, as seen on the right-hand side of Table 2–1.

Experimental Studies

The first of the explanatory study designs is the *experimental* strategy, which is familiar to most of us from undergraduate chemistry or psychology. In medical research it travels under the aliases of the controlled trial, clinical trial, healthcare trial, or intervention trial. The primary feature that distinguishes the trial from other explanatory studies is the active intervention of the investigator. For example, the researcher gives an antidepressant medication to one group of volunteers and a placebo to another group; or one-half of a medical-school class is selected to receive a new self-instructional package on anemia while the other half gets a lecture; or patients in a practice are randomly assigned to a physician or to a nurse practitioner for care. In each case, the researcher who is testing the efficacy of the method is able to exercise control by assigning subjects to medications, lectures, or nurse practitioners. Figure 2–1 illustrates the general outline of the controlled trial. It is an important form of study design and will be dealt with in more detail later.

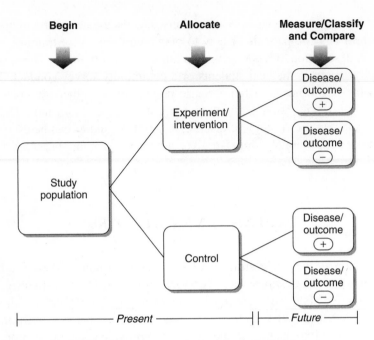

FIGURE 2–1. Experimental, or controlled trial, design.

Observational Studies

Observational studies also utilize comparisons to examine and explain medical mysteries. They often evolve from simple associations discovered in the course of daily experience that appear to link health outcomes with factors in our environment—the high rate of heart disease in those who eat large amounts of animal fat compared with those who are vegetarians, for example. However, unlike the experimental design, the observational study relegates researchers to the role of bystanders. They examine the natural course of health events, gather data about subjects, and classify and sort the data. By the strategy of making comparisons, they then try to provide insights into the cause of diseases.

The plethora of terms at the beginning of this chapter notwithstanding, there is really only a limited number of ways of approaching an observational study. We can start by studying individuals who already have a particular disease or outcome (patients with colon cancer or who have low satisfaction with medical care, or doctors who have become surgeons) and search for some risks or factors in their past that may explain the outcome. Figure 2–2 outlines this case-control approach. Alternatively, we can begin

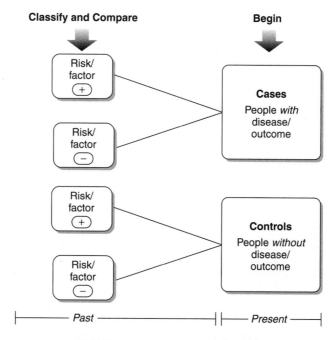

FIGURE 2–2. Case-control design.

with a group of individuals who do not yet have the outcome of interest, examine and classify them by characteristics we think might be related to the outcome, and follow-up to see which patients develop disease (see Figure 2–3).

A. Case-Control Design: We begin with the outcome—such as colon cancer, low patient satisfaction, or surgical specialty—and look for features of people who share that outcome. Do they eat too little fiber, spend more time in the waiting room, or have exceptionally high personal motivation when compared with people who do not have cancer, are not dissatisfied, or are not surgeons? If differences in frequencies of the characteristics between the cases and the comparison group are found, we have taken a positive step toward explaining the outcome. We will call this the *case-control* approach, although it should be clear from the examples used that the term *case* is used broadly to define an individual who already has the outcome of interest. That outcome need not be a medical disease. The term *case control* does convey the major activity of the design: that we begin at the end—with people who have the outcome—and compare their

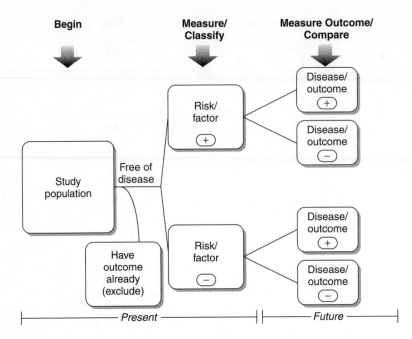

FIGURE 2–3. Follow-up design.

exposures or habits of the past with subjects who do not have that outcome (see Figure 2–2).

B. Follow-Up Design: In this approach we start with people who have not yet experienced the outcome: healthy people, new registrants in a practice, or third-year medical students. Characteristics of the group, such as diet, waiting time, or motivation, are measured and cataloged, and the researcher sits back and watches for cancer, dissatisfaction, or choice of medical specialty to develop. Again, using comparisons such as the rate of dissatisfaction among patients who wait against those who are seen promptly, the researcher casts light on possible causes of the outcome. This approach is most commonly referred to as the *cohort,* or *follow-up,* design because it begins with a cohort or group and follows it until the outcome appears (see Figure 2–3).

C. Cross-Sectional Design: A third variation on the observational study is the *cross-sectional* approach. A blend of the two strategies just discussed, the cross-sectional design begins with a population or cohort and makes simultaneous assessments of outcomes, descriptive features, and potential predictors. This "slice-in-time design" is also referred to as a *prevalence survey,* because its population basis makes it possible to estimate the frequency of disease within a group (see Figure 2–4). The approach can be used for explanatory purposes or in giving a descriptive account of an outcome or disease. For example, a community survey of blood lead levels in young children identifies the extent (prevalence) of lead poisoning in the community and assesses the need for medical services. If information is obtained on the children's environments, the cause of elevated blood lead levels can also be evaluated. Another example is a national telephone survey of U.S. adults that compares the use of medical services, such as routine checkups and preventive services according to health insurance status.

A Concocted Example

For purposes of illustration, we can take a single example and try out each of the major explanatory approaches. To give us a working terminology,

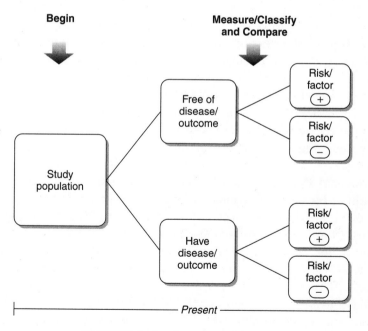

FIGURE 2–4. Cross-sectional design.

we will call them case-control, follow-up, cross-sectional, and intervention trial designs.

A. The Problem: During the past few years of practice, we have made a fascinating clinical observation. In talking to patients who have poor visual acuity and wear glasses, we have noted that their diets seem to be remarkably deficient in carrots. Now everyone knows that the carotenes that give carrots their lovely orange glow are essential for the formation of rhodopsin, a retinal pigment associated with good night vision, but it appears we are onto the illuminating discovery that previously unappreciated components of carrots may actually aid visual acuity. In fact, our first informal survey revealed that of 5 bespectacled patients queried, all admitted to a singular disinterest in carrots. The question is how to pursue this exciting hunch and create an explanatory study that will substantiate our hypothesis that an association exists between good vision and carrot consumption.

B. Case-Control Design: We begin by collecting 100 of our spectacle-wearing patients to represent the cases. They already have the outcome—poor visual acuity. As a comparison or control group, we identify another 100 individuals—patients who are generally like our first group except that they enjoy 20/20 vision. We then proceed to ask each of these 200 people to give us an exhaustive accounting of their dietary habits over recent years, paying particular attention to their consumption of carrots. Our hope will be that a conspicuous difference in carrot eating will be found between those with good and those with poor vision. If patients with poor vision are well below the comparison group with respect to carrot intake, we will have evidence to support the link between carrots and eyesight. Figure 2–5 reflects all this.

C. Follow-Up Design: Figure 2–6 shows how our example might look as a follow-up study. All patients who enter the practice will be given a test for visual acuity. Subjects who already have poor acuity will be dropped from further consideration. They already have the outcome. For the remainder, those with good vision, dietary records will be maintained so that we will have an accurate account of the carrot intake of all our subjects. These people will be followed up for the next 10 years, and at the end of that time everyone's vision will be retested. Armed with information on carrot consumption with which to classify subjects, we will be able to compare the vision status of patients with high intake with that of

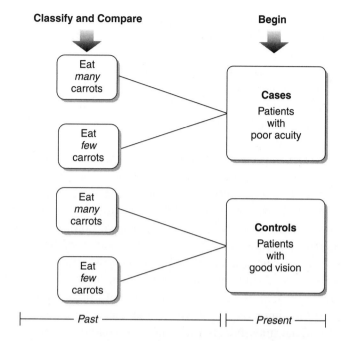

FIGURE 2–5. Case-control design: An illustration.

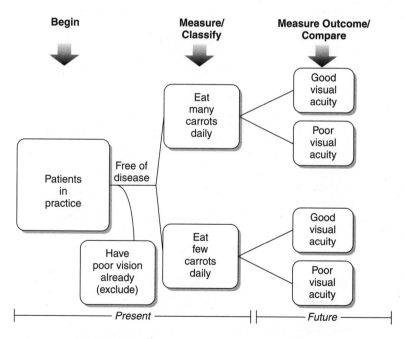

FIGURE 2–6. Follow-up design: An illustration.

patients who eat few or no carrots at all. If carrot eaters see better than those who eschew the orange roots, our hypothesis will be supported. It should be emphasized that the follow-up design just described is an observational rather than an experimental study, even though as investigators we seemed to be assuming a very active role. We examined eyesight and counted carrots, but we never told our patients how many carrots they should eat. That was left to nature.

D. Cross-Sectional Design: On the way to performing our follow-up study, we dismissed the portion of our population who were screened and found lacking in visual acuity. We could have gained some information from this group, however. Had we taken the trouble to ask them about their current carrot-eating habits, we could have compared their intake with the carrot consumption of patients with good eyesight. This slice of information from our practice would be a cross-sectional study: Do patients with good vision eat more carrots than those with poor vision? (see Figure 2–7). As in the case-control study, information on diet is from the past, albeit the immediate past. Unlike the case-control design, however, the cross-sectional study begins with a large population instead of selected

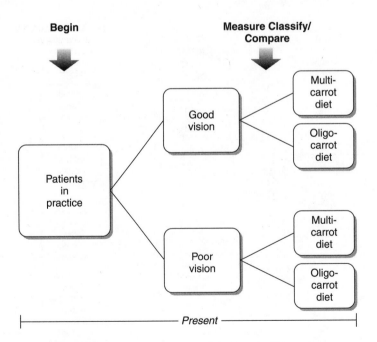

FIGURE 2–7. Cross-sectional design: An illustration.

cases. Classifying patients by both carrot consumption and vision, we learn the prevalence of low acuity in the practice and get an estimate of the role that carrot eating plays in deficient vision.

E. Intervention Trial Design: We again begin with a group of patients who are free of the outcome, that is, have good vision (see Figure 2–8). We divide our population into two groups. To the first we offer a special diet including everything from carrot daiquiris to carrot cake. In the diet of the second group, carrots and their by-products are avoided.

During the months and years that follow, we diligently perform vision examinations to see how our two groups fare and ultimately compare the high- and low-carrot-diet groups with respect to vision outcomes.

Each of these strategies has a distinctive flavor. The case-control format has an economy about it, but one can sense difficulties in retrieving information from the past and in finding proper groups to compare. The follow-up and intervention trial designs allow better planning and control but require ongoing diligence to keep track of subjects and see that people stay on their diets. We will examine the advantages of the different methodologies as well as explore their limitations and tribulations in the next few chapters.

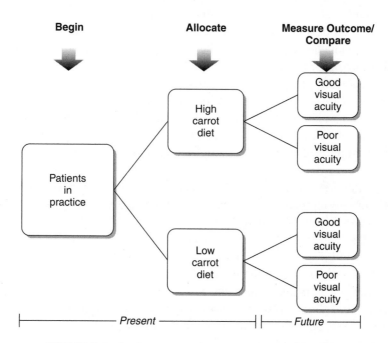

FIGURE 2–8. Experimental, or intervention trial, design.

MORE CONFUSING TERMINOLOGY

Identifying study designs can be a perplexing business. Even people who ought to know better occasionally get caught with their terms in a tangle. Bits of jargon that are particularly troublesome are the duos: cases and controls and prospective and retrospective. The ambiguous use of these terms accounts for considerable confusion.

Prospective & Retrospective

Among the confusing terms encountered in descriptions of medical studies are references to prospective and retrospective designs. It does not take an etymologist to tell you that these two words describe a relationship to time—looking forward in time and looking backward. Unfortunately, in common medical usage they have also come to be synonyms for design structures. Studies we call case-control designs are also known as retrospective studies; those that we designate as cohort, or follow-up, studies are also referred to as prospective studies.

Time can be a bugbear unless readers keep the time frame in which a study is conducted separate from the strategy of comparison that is being used. *Retrospective studies* begin and end in the present but involve a major backward glance to collect information about events that occurred in the past. *Prospective studies* also begin in the present but march forward, collecting data about a population whose outcome lies in the future. But these two terms do not offer sufficient precision about the strategy of the study. It should be clear, for example, that both the controlled trial and the follow-up design proceed in a prospective, forward fashion. Both these strategies begin with a population, gather measurements, and watch for developments in the future, but conceptually, experimental versus observational strategies are different.

Similarly, the notion that any study using data that are collected retrospectively falls into the case-control category is misleading. One design utilizes the follow-up technique but does it using information from the past. This strategy labors under the awkward designation of *retrospective follow-up, historical prospective,* or *retrospective cohort* design. The key to the success of this approach (as diagrammed in Figure 2–9) is the availability of carefully kept records from the past.

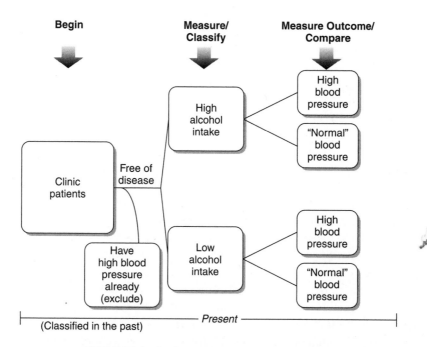

FIGURE 2–9. Retrospective follow-up design.

Researchers wishing to examine the relationship between alcohol consumption and development of high blood pressure might need to wait 20 years before high blood pressure develops in patients they have screened and classified with respect to alcohol consumption. If, however, they can find medical records that document the drinking habits and blood pressures of people 15–20 years ago, they can greatly condense the time frame of the study. They select a cohort of people whose alcohol consumption was conscientiously recorded in the past, follow them up to the present by measuring current blood pressures, and produce a *retrospective follow-up* study. No waiting is required for disease to develop, and data are collected prior to the onset of illness and so are not susceptible to faulty memories.

Cases & Controls

What are we to make of an article that gives itself simultaneous billing as a "long-term case-control study" and an account of the "natural history of bacteriuria in schoolgirls?"[4] Pause and reflect. A study tracking the natural history of something ought to be following up on subjects with certain characteristics for a period of time to see what happens to them. This does not sound like a case-control design, which starts with people who have an outcome and tries to discover relevant past habits. Sure enough, in this study the investigators evaluated 60 schoolgirls who were found through a screening program to have bacteriuria, then reexamined them periodically for several years to determine the ones in whom renal complications developed. Complication rates for girls who had bacteriuria were found to be substantially higher when compared with rates for a group of girls who were without infections. A perfect example of a follow-up study!

The confusion arises because of the use of the term "case" to describe girls who have bacteriuria. They are indeed cases as the clinician uses the term—to identify patients who have a disease or health condition. They are not cases, however, in the sense the researcher uses the term—to define a group with an outcome that will serve as a starting point for a comparative study. Bacteriuria is not the outcome of this observational study. The outcome is chronic renal disease. Bacteriuria is a characteristic shared by a portion of the initial cohort of schoolgirls that we wish to follow up. At the same time, "controls" as used in this paper are really a subset of girls from a larger population who were screened for urinary tract infection and found free of bacteriuria. They are followed forward in time for comparative purposes and assessed for renal complications. They are not the foils in a case-control design.

Another study, billing itself as a "prospective case-control study," describes the role of astroviruses in acute diarrhea among hospitalized children.[5] It does not qualify as a case-control study either. In the course of their research, the investigators cultured the stools of children hospitalized with diarrhea. Because many pathogens isolated inhabit the gastrointestinal tract of normal children in a nonpathogenic state, a group of children admitted to the hospital for conditions other than diarrhea was included for comparison. These control children had stool cultures obtained concurrent with their admissions, as did the youngsters with diarrhea. Think for a moment. The structure of this study is neither looking backward to determine exposures of the past that might lead to conditions of the present, nor are these children being followed up over time to assess outcomes in the future. It is really a cross-sectional design. Both cases and controls are measured and classified at the time of their illness for factors (in this case, viruses) that might be related to their condition.

When researchers find that astrovirus is present in 7% of children with diarrhea but in none without diarrhea, they have grounds for believing the virus may be responsible for the diarrhea. The terminology is confusing but the findings quite useful.

To quibble with Gertrude Stein a bit—a case is not a case is not a case. Sometimes a case is a subject in a specific explanatory strategy who has been chosen because she has the outcome under study—bacteriuria, low satisfaction, or poor visual acuity. Sometimes that same bacteriuria, low satisfaction, or poor visual acuity is the starting point of the study, and groups of cases that share a characteristic are watched for development of outcomes, such as renal failure, broken appointments, or traffic accidents. Readers must avoid the temptation to classify every article that refers to cases and controls as a case-control study. It may be a follow-up or experimental design.

SUMMARY

Having gone through the strenuous exercise of pinning a label on the structure of a study, what reward can we expect for the effort? The next three chapters will burrow deeper into the problems of design and, it is hoped, will come out with useful advice for assessing the strengths and weaknesses of common designs. To place the study into a methodological category, ask the following questions:

1. Is the design a descriptive or explanatory effort? Is the author simply detailing an experience with cases, practices, or treatments, or making comparisons in hopes of establishing etiologies or evaluating interventions?

2. If comparisons are being made, is the investigator observing the course of events, or creating an experiment by assigning subjects to receive a pill, an exercise program, or a piece of health advice?

3. If the design is observational, are patients who already have a disease or outcome compared with unaffected controls for preexisting characteristics? Or do investigators classify and follow a cohort of subjects for development of the outcome or effect of interest?

REFERENCES

1. Lilienfeld DE: Definitions of epidemiology. Am J Epidemiol 1978;107:87.
2. Heberden W: Commentaries on the history and cure of diseases. In: Willius FA, Keys TE (editors): *Classics of Cardiology,* Vol. 1. Dover Publications, 1961.
3. Hymes KB et al: Kaposi's sarcoma in homosexual men: A report of eight cases. Lancet 1981;2:598.
4. Gillenwater JY, Harrison RB, Kunin CM: Natural history of bacteriuria in schoolgirls: A long-term case-control study. N Engl J Med 1979;301:396.
5. Dennehy PH et al: A prospective case-control study of the role of astrovirus in acute diarrhea among hospitalized young children. J Infect Dis 2001;184(1):10.

CHAPTER THREE

Study Design: The Case-Control Approach

. . . you yourself sir, should be as old as I am if, like a crab, you could go backward

HAMLET, ACT II, SCENE II

It is not so many years since case-control studies were much maligned. A particularly bright remark referencing Dr. Rasputin's work on hemophilia would be rebuffed by the put-down, "Of course those were retrospective studies." The implication is clear. A retrospective or case-control design is a crude masquerade for a research study. Some continue to argue that satisfactory solutions to research questions can never be obtained through the case-control methodology because there are insurmountable problems in going backward.

It is well to clear our heads now of sweeping prejudices against the case-control design. For, although the method falls prey to a number of difficulties, it has become standard fare. With the costs and time required to perform long-term, follow-up studies on large populations, the case-control design has clear efficiencies to offer. . There are several attractive features that should be recognized before we start considering its tender points.

ADVANTAGES OF THE CASE-CONTROL DESIGN

The case-control design is ideally suited for initial, explanatory ventures. As we have seen with the observations on Kaposi's sarcoma[1] or the example of carrots and vision, many important medical discoveries begin with a clinical observation or hunch. An unusual clustering of cases of cancer is noted, a surprising side effect is observed following the use of an antibiotic, many children with learning disabilities are reported to have been formula fed as infants. The handiest way to see if these hunches lead to valid discoveries is to make some quick comparisons with subjects who are readily at hand. Are patients with mesothelioma more likely to have been exposed to asbestos than a comparison group? Is there a difference in the history of breast and bottle feeding between children with learning disabilities and those who perform well in school? The case-control design is ideal for trying these hypotheses. It is very *efficient.* Since our novel observations generally begin with patients who have experienced the unusual disease or side effect, collecting cases is relatively easy. Hospitals and outpatient clinics are replete with patients who already have diseases or outcomes we may wish to study. We need not wait years for the outcome to develop or expend great energy tracking down subjects who require follow-up.

Another widely advertised advantage of the case-control design is its *utility for studying rare diseases.* This point certainly appears to have merit, since even diseases we think of as common occur relatively infrequently. The annual incidence of breast cancer, for example, is about 1 per 1000 women; only about 1 in 100 men between 50 and 59 years of age will have a heart attack each year. This means that to perform follow-up studies, extremely large populations must be monitored to supply even a handful of cases.

The case-control approach is also conducive to voyages into the uncharted waters of disease etiology. To this end, in anticipation of future explorations, large data banks have been collected detailing all sorts of information on patients from their habits of alcohol consumption to their zoonotic afflictions. Rather than beginning with a hunch they wish to test, investigators engage in "hypothesis generation" or what some disparage as "data dredging" or "fishing."[2] Patients with a disease such as endometrial cancer are culled from the database, and a list of their behavioral and pharmacological exposures is compared to the exposure frequencies of a control group selected from the same database. Many comparisons are made, and sometimes, by virtue of persistence and force of numbers, associations between a medication or habit and the disease are discovered.

PROBLEMS OF CASE-CONTROL DESIGNS

The objective of the case-control design is to identify causes of a disease or other outcomes. The strategy is to compare the frequency of a risk factor among those who are afflicted compared with those who are not. All other things being equal (which is not always the case), differential rates of exposure point to etiology. If dissatisfied patients wait twice as long in the waiting room as those who are pleased with their care, or people with colon cancer eat half as much fiber as those without cancer, we have evidence that increased waiting time and low-fiber diets may be responsible for the adverse outcomes. Essential to the validity of case-control designs is the appropriate selection of cases and controls, and the adequacy and comparability of the exposure data obtained. We will look at these issues in turn.

Selection of Cases

A. Sample Selection: The choice of cases can create difficulties if those sampled do not represent the larger population of those who have the outcome. A highly screened sample, such as patients admitted to a referral hospital, may not offer an accurate reflection of the broader world of patients with rheumatoid arthritis or type1 diabetes.

A case-control study that was designed to discover whether maternal smoking and alcohol consumption during pregnancy predispose infants to febrile seizures illustrates this problem.[3] Febrile seizure cases in this endeavor were identified primarily through emergency room log books from 20 western Washington hospitals. For each childhood seizure case, a control was recruited, using birth records of infants born at the same hospital during the same week. When control candidates could not be contacted or declined participation, investigators returned to the birth registries and identified another child born as proximate to the case as possible. Telephone interviews were conducted with mothers of both groups. Prenatal histories of health habits, including use of alcohol and tobacco during pregnancy, were obtained. Results indicated that mothers of infants who had seizures were more likely to have smoked cigarettes and consumed alcohol during pregnancy than mothers in the comparison (control) group. Babies born to the women in the case group were twice as likely as control group infants to experience febrile seizures—further evidence for the adverse consequences of smoking and drinking during pregnancy. However, a critical commentary published with this report suggests that bias may have crept in when cases were chosen.[4] The critique points out that many children with febrile seizures are not seen in emergency rooms. Those who do seek emergency room care are often from families without regular physicians, families who may be less health conscious in other health behaviors, such as smoking and drinking. They are not likely to be representative of the broader population of children from which controls were selected. Estimates of maternal alcohol and tobacco use would thus be spuriously high and the estimates of seizure risk associated with these behaviors exaggerated.

It is also important that cases not be identified *because* of their exposure. If the knowledge that a subject has a potential risk factor prompts diagnosis of the disease or outcome, study validity may be jeopardized. The editors of the *Journal of the American Medical Association* provided an illustration when they published 2 papers with differing views on the role of tampons in the etiology of an illness that made the headlines in the late 1970s. Toxic shock syndrome (TSS) occurred in a number of young women who suddenly developed high fever, progressive skin rash, and falling blood pressure. Most were menstruating at the time. The first paper came from the Centers for Disease Control and Prevention (CDC) and was one of several case-control studies that looked for risk factors for TSS.[5] Using the classic case-control approach, investigators identified patients whose episodes of TSS had been reported to the CDC. The 50 women selected were asked to identify 3 acquaintances of approximately the same age who lived in the same geographic area. These friends formed a control group. Cases and controls were interviewed by telephone and asked to identify the type of "menstrual device" used during the month in which the woman became ill. All 50 of the selected cases but only 125 of 150 controls had used tampons during their menstrual period. This finding created a significant association between tampon use and the development of TSS.

In the same issue of the journal, a group from Yale University critically reviewed publications that linked toxic shock and tampon use[6] and noted that bias might have occurred because of the way cases were identified.

Early reports linking the syndrome to menstruation and possibly to tampon use had received wide publicity by the time several of the research studies had begun. A *diagnostic bias* might have occurred if patients with equivocal criteria for TSS were given the diagnosis because they were known to be menstruating and using tampons. The critics cited an example where a woman whose symptoms were, in fact, most suggestive of *Shigella* enteritis was diagnosed as TSS for just such reasons. *Reporting bias* might also be present and work in a similar fashion. Because of the publicity implicating menstruation and tampon use as risks for TSS, physicians might have been more likely to report an episode to the CDC if the patient's history was positive for these two features. As it turned out, the findings of the case-control studies linking TSS to tampon use were supported by other work. Still, the potential for biases deserves consideration.

B. Case Definitions: Cases need to be carefully defined. Is the author talking about a clearly delineated, homogeneous problem? Is a single outcome being considered, or are multiple, related conditions, which might have different etiologies, being inappropriately lumped together? No one would consider a case-control study that combined cases of leukemia, Wilms tumor, and colorectal cancer in a single "cancer" category.

If the sample of cases is diluted by the unwitting inclusion of subjects who do not truly have the disease or outcome of interest, a true association between the exposure and disease may be missed. A large, national case-control study of a devastating childhood illness known as Reye syndrome provides an illustration. Named after the Australian pathologist who first described it, the condition is marked by a fulminate, frequently fatal encephalopathy that comes in the wake of an apparently nonthreatening illness such as chicken pox or influenza. In the large U.S. Public Health Service study that identified a relationship between Reye syndrome and aspirin use, 70 pediatric referral centers were enlisted to identify this unusual but life-threatening condition.[7] Because the early symptoms of the disease—a mild respiratory or gastrointestinal illness—might be confused with other conditions, investigators were careful to include as cases only subjects who met rigorous criteria and passed review of a physician panel. As it happened, 53 patients were reported through the hospital network, but only 27 met the standards as bona fide cases of Reye syndrome and were included in the final study. It is easy to imagine that the medication histories of the 26 excluded might have been dissimilar. So, although it appears that something was lost by cutting the number of study cases in half, the increased confidence that a homogeneous disease entity was being evaluated more than compensates. Had the other 26 reported "cases" been included, overall exposure frequencies to aspirin would likely have been less than the 96% that was found, and the strong association linking the drug and the disease would have been substantially reduced.

Selection of Controls

The choice of an appropriate control group is also a challenging proposition. The idea, of course, is to find a group of individuals who come from the same general population as cases but who do not have heart disease, bronchitis, or low satisfaction, for example. Our need is to derive an estimate of "general" rates of exposure to high-fat diets, secondhand smoke, or prolonged waiting room time. Finding a group that represents this "general population" is more difficult than one might think. The choice of controls can bias results by selectively including subjects who either underestimate or overestimate exposures.

One commonly utilized source of control subjects that is notorious for creating this dilemma is the hospital. Because patients with serious diseases are easy to locate in hospitals, selecting controls from the same hospital population is not only convenient but sensible. Subjects in the same facility are likely to come from the same community and have similar access to the health system. When investigators from Boston explored the relationship between coffee consumption and cancer of the pancreas, they found histories of higher coffee intake among cancer patients than among controls.[8] Cases of pancreatic cancer were obtained from 11 large metropolitan hospitals. Controls were selected from patients who were under the care of the same physician in the same hospital as cases. It turned out that "because of the nature of practices of many of the physicians, patients with gastroenterologic conditions were probably overrepresented in relation to a general hospital population."[8] These included patients with hernia, colitis, enteritis, diverticulitis, and a variety of other conditions. The authors themselves expressed concern that the coffee-drinking habits of such a control group might not represent those of the population at large. Patients with gastroenterological problems may not drink much coffee, either because it worsens their condition or because their doctors admonished them against coffee use. If coffee intake by controls is spuriously low, that of cancer patients appears elevated in comparison, and a false association between coffee and pancreatic cancer results.

Silverman et al[9] studied the prevalence of coffee drinking among hospitalized and population-based groups. Using data from a national study conducted in the Detroit area, they found that the pattern of coffee drinking among all hospitalized patients was similar to that in the overall population. However, in the subgroup of patients with digestive disorders, the number of cups of coffee taken per day was significantly lower. Only 55% of hospitalized patients with gastrointestinal problems drank 2 or more cups of coffee per day compared with 73% of population controls. The difference in coffee-drinking habits of patients with pancreatic cancer and controls may thus not be due to a link between the beverage and the disease but rather to the selection of a control group with an unusually low prevalence of the risk factor.

An inappropriate control group can have the opposite effect and obscure an important link between a disease and its cause. Suppose, for example, that hospitalized patients who have had heart attacks are questioned regarding their smoking habits. If the reports of these patients are compared with those of other, general hospital patients, the connection between smoking and heart disease could be lost. Many hospitalized patients have other smoking-related diseases, such as emphysema, bronchitis, or lung cancer. They may admit to cigarette usage every bit as high as that of heart disease patients.

Alleviating Control-Group Problems

A. Multiple Controls: One approach to warding off the demons of control selection is to employ more than one control group. Multiple control groups can offer independent estimates of exposure among different samples of noncases and substantially strengthen a study's findings. The Public Health Service study of Reye syndrome and medications is a creative illustration.[7] Rather than settle for a single control group, researchers enlisted subjects to represent 4 different populations. All controls were children of approximately the same age as case subjects. All had recently had a respiratory or gastrointestinal illness. But because investigators were concerned about the selective forces that place some children with respiratory illness in hospitals while others remain at home and the relevance that this might have to medication use, they chose a spectrum of control subjects.

Children who are patients in referral centers are likely to have illnesses that are comparable in severity to Reye syndrome and so make logical controls. But this group may overrepresent children with chronic illnesses, who may take more medications than a typical child or may have been instructed to avoid certain drugs. Emergency room patients constituted another group. Such sick children are easy to locate and have antecedent illnesses that are more like those of the cases in severity, but they have a lower burden of chronic disease. Two other groups were obtained to offer a picture of more general medication use, one from among children attending the same school or day care center as the case and the other from a random-digit-dialing telephone survey. These children were clearly much less severely ill than Reye syndrome cases. With 4 control groups, 4 estimates of "general" medication use were available.

Results were dramatic. Ninety-six percent of Reye syndrome patients reported use of salicylates, compared with only 40% of emergency room controls, 44% of school controls, and 35% of random-digit-dialing telephone controls (see Table 3–1). Only 27% of hospital controls had been given salicylates. The relatively consistent rate of control-group exposure using these very different populations strengthens one's confidence that the exposures of cases and controls were truly different. Rates of medications other than salicylates were also tallied and found to be similar across case and control groups. An exception was acetaminophen, an analgesic/antipyretic substitute for aspirin, where usage was considerably higher for controls than cases (see Table 3–1). All this serves to further enhance the association between salicylate use and Reye syndrome.

B. Community Controls: Community controls are commonly used to gain more accurate estimates of exposure among the non-ill for comparison purposes. They frequently come from the neighborhoods or social groups to which the cases belong. These controls can also be recruited through random community surveys conducted by mail or telephone.

In a paper that attempted to determine environmental and social features that distinguished children seen in a psychiatric outpatient clinic from other children, a sample of children seen in several psychiatric outpatient facilities was contrasted with 2 control groups.[10] The first was a hospital control group that consisted of children from the pediatric clinic, children from the ophthalmology clinic, and children who had had an appendectomy or tonsillectomy. The second group came from the same neighborhood as the cases but was not part of an identified hospital or clinic population. The authors queried parents of the children in each of these 3 groups about a host of factors, ranging from whether the child had nightmares and temper tantrums to the marital relationship of the parents, the child's progress in school, and whether or not the child was spanked.

TABLE 3–1
Medication exposures of Reye's syndrome cases and 4 control groups

Medication	Cases (n = 27)	Controls[a] Inpatient (n = 22)	ER (n = 30)	School (n = 45)	Community (n = 43)	Total (n = 140)
Acetaminophen	26.9	77.3	90.0	91.1	81.4	85.7
Chlorpheniramine	22.2	22.7	23.3	20.0	37.2	26.4
Phenylephrine	14.8	22.7	6.7	20.0	20.9	17.9
Pseudoephedrine	29.6	31.8	16.7	26.7	48.8	32.1
Salicylates/aspirin	96.3	27.3	40.0	44.4	34.9	37.9

[a]Controls obtained from hospital inpatient and emergency rooms (ER), schools, and random-digit-dialing telephone survey (Community). Modified, with permission, from Hurwitz et al.[7]

Not surprisingly, children from the psychiatric clinic showed more problem behaviors and disrupted families than control children. However, a "striking and unexpected finding was the difference between the hospital control and community control [patients]." Factors such as parental loss, fears, temper tantrums, nightmares, and reports of maladjustment at school occurred much more frequently among control children chosen from the clinics than among those taken from the neighborhood. The difference was seen despite the intentional selection of hospital controls who had minor illnesses and surgical procedures. It suggests that children who get into the medical system, regardless of the reason, have characteristics that differ from those of a group of community kids.

The hazard in using community controls lies not in the source but in the sampling. It is critical that community subjects who are located through surveys and who agree to participate in the study present a representative risk profile. Individuals without telephones cannot be included in a random-digit-dialing survey. Employed people may not be at home if contact is attempted during working hours. Some may simply find participation too onerous, too threatening, or too unimportant. If these folks have different habits, beliefs, and behaviors from individuals who are successfully contacted and agree to serve as control subjects, the community is not being reflected accurately.

A case-control study designed to evaluate a possible link between hemorrhagic stroke in relatively young adults and use of medications containing the decongestant/appetite suppressant, phenylpropanolamine (PPA), employed random-digit-dialing to find subjects to compare with patients who had suffered strokes.[11] For each control subject enrolled, the investigative team needed to make on average 150 phone calls. Even though much of the dialing did not result in contact with a household, a low yield invites the question whether participating control subjects accurately represent the community from which the cases come. When stroke patients and controls were compared, the cases had, indeed, consumed more PPA. However, the groups differed in a variety of other ways as well. Controls were better educated, smoked less, were less often hypertensive, and had lower rates of alcohol and cocaine use. The list of dissimilarities suggests that the two samples may differ in a variety of ways. There may be factors other than the use of PPA that are responsible for strokes.

C. Matching: One way of dealing with factors that may confuse the comparison between cases and controls is to employ a technique known as *matching.* This term is frequently encountered in descriptions of study methods. It means that investigators have made an effort to select control subjects who share particular characteristics with the cases. Matching has a specific purpose. It improves the efficiency of a study by keeping constant or controlling factors that are known to be related to the outcome and may confuse results if they occur disproportionately in the groups that are being compared.

Suppose we wish to evaluate a hunch we have developed that cigar smoking causes people to lose their hair. To study this question in the case-control mode, we first select a group of balding patients from the dermatology clinic—patients who are undergoing a new hair-implantation procedure. As soon as they feel up to wrinkling their brows, we quiz them about their past habits, making special note of cigar smoking. We then need to ask the same questions of a comparison group. A little thought suggests that trotting down the hallway to the pediatric clinic would be unwise. The youngsters there, although clinic patients, bear little resemblance to the patients undergoing hair transplants. The obvious difference, age, is an important one because it is related to the habit and the outcome. Cigar smoking is an activity that increases with age; so does baldness. One would expect a higher rate of cigar smoking among the dermatology clinic patients because they are older, not because cigars cause baldness. We would be ill advised to advertise a link between stogie puffing and alopecia without some way of accounting for the role of age.

Matching reduces competing explanations for the outcome in question. If we selected age-matched controls to compare with our bald patients— that is, if we chose subjects who were close in age to our cases—we would eliminate or control any confusion about whether it is really smoking or just age that is related to hair loss. If we still found higher smoking rates among cases, it would not be because of differential ages in the groups. This kind of matching may be done on a case-by-case basis, where each bald patient is matched with a hairy subject who is within 1 or 2 years of being the same age. It may also be accomplished in groups, where both cases and controls are chosen from patients who fall within a specified age range. Age is probably the most commonly matched variable because it is related to so many habits and diseases that come under study. Sex, race, and socioeconomic status are other commonly used variables, but matching may be carried out on any factor, from apple-cider drinking to exposure to zinc smelters.

Creative use of matching was achieved by researchers investigating the role of alcohol use in fatal and serious bicycle injuries.[12] Cases of 124 Maryland cyclists, 15 years and older, who were fatally injured or required hospitalization and had blood alcohol concentrations obtained were used. So far, so good. But where does one find appropriate controls? The challenge is not simply to find injured subjects, but to find those who also ride bicycles and have alcohol use data available. Such controls are not typically found sitting in hospital or clinic waiting rooms. So investigators went to the field to find their comparison subjects. For each case, interviewers traveled to the location where the injury occurred at the same time of day, on the same day of the week and month. They stopped passing bicyclists and requested a brief interview and breath sample for alcohol. Such ingenious matching creates a control group that is like the population from which the cases arise. In fact, the 2 groups look quite similar when their demographic features are displayed (see Table 3–2). When we learn that alcohol was used by 24% of fatal cases, 9% of nonfatal cases, and only 3% of controls,

TABLE 3–2

Alcohol and bicycle injury: Selected characteristics of cases and controls

Characteristics	% of cases ($n = 124$)	Controls ($n = 342$)
Sex		
Men	83.1	81.9
Women	16.1	18.1
Age, years		
15–19	23.4	17.0
20–29	25.0	23.7
30–39	21.0	29.5
40–49	16.9	17.8
50–59	8.1	8.8
≥60	5.6	3.2
Race		
White	73.4	67.3
Black	22.6	29.8
Other	4.0	2.9
Marital status		
Never married	61.5	54.7
Married	32.3	32.2
Other	6.3	13.2

Modified, with permission, from Li et al.[12]

we are encouraged that it is alcohol rather than some risk of the site, season, or time of day that is responsible for the serious injuries.

D. Overmatching: Matching is a lovely technique for creating order in the world. However, there is a price to be paid for matching. An investigator can overmatch. Matching equalizes the occurrence of a factor in the groups that are being compared; therefore, once cases and controls are matched by age, sex, or whatever, these factors can no longer be evaluated as possible etiologic agents. As an obvious example, suppose we are fledgling hematologists, unencumbered by previous knowledge about causes of anemia. We have discovered a group of patients with severe anemia who have unusual, sickle-shaped red blood cells in their blood smears. In an attempt to learn more about the etiology of this disease, we devise a clever case-control, observational study in which we match patients who have anemia with nonanemic medical patients of the same age, race, and sex. We note in passing that the cases all happen to be Black and, therefore, we select only Blacks as control patients. We have overmatched. By matching for race, we have lost our ability to show that sickle cell anemia has a genetic basis as reflected by differential occurrence in Whites and Blacks.

Nor does matching guarantee that groups being compared are balanced. Investigators in the PPA study[11] selected control subjects who were matched to cases by age, race, and sex. The groups still turned out to be disturbingly dissimilar.

E. Case-Crossover Design: A variant on the case-control study that readers may encounter is the *case-crossover* design. In this approach, *each case becomes his or her own control.* Sounds improbable. How can someone be both with and without the outcome or disease of interest? It is easy if the outcome is a discrete occurrence associated with a transient exposure. Motor vehicle collisions and cellular telephone use are an example.

In an attempt to ascertain whether drivers distracted by cell phones were likely to be involved in auto collisions, 2 Canadian investigators queried almost 700 drivers who had been in a collision and had a cell phone.[13] Using police records, phone logs, and interviews, they ascertained that 24% of the drivers had been talking on their phones in the 10 minutes preceding the collision. But is that more or less than one would expect? How does one find an appropriate comparison group? Should one use other drivers who do not have cell phones, or drivers who have them but were not in a collision? It is difficult to decide on an appropriate comparison for this particular group of cases.

To solve the problem, investigators elected to use cases as their own controls, picking the same time period as the day before the collision as a reference point. Only 5% of subjects had used their phones at the same time period on the previous day. After making adjustments for the fact that about one-third of cases were not driving the day before the collision, researchers calculated that cell phone use was associated with a fourfold increased likelihood of collision. Because cases served as their own controls, factors such as age, socioeconomic status, and employment, that might have confused the association between cell phone use and collision were eliminated.

The case-crossover design has been used to evaluate possible precipitating events for acute myocardial infarction, the relation between alcohol use and injuries, and exposure to beta-agonist drugs and asthma attacks. It has the obvious advantages of eliminating the problems of searching for controls who mirror cases except for the disease or outcome. The ability to sample other periods of time before a critical event—the day before, last week, last month—as well as to employ more traditional comparison subjects means that multiple estimates of control data are possible.

Exposure Information

It is critical to acquire accurate exposure data on cases and controls. If information collected from the 2 groups is not of comparable quality, we are in for trouble. Since exposure data are assembled after outcomes are known, it is not difficult to imagine that such knowledge might influence the gathering of information. Both subjects and investigators may fall prey to bias that occurs when one looks backward.

A. Subject Bias: Many case-control studies rely on information supplied by the subjects themselves. However, case and comparison subjects are apt to have considered the past rather differently. People who have unpleasant diseases are likely to have scrutinized past events with much greater vigor than nondiseased individuals. It is human nature to seek explanations for tragedies. So it should not surprise us that people who are beleaguered by illness or unpleasant outcomes have contemplated deeply what caused their problem and may have an overly detailed, even distorted picture of the past. The phenomenon is known as *selective recall, reporting*, or *recall bias*, and is accentuated when subjects already hold beliefs about the cause of their disease.

Case-control studies that query patients about prior sun exposure as a potential cause of malignant melanoma offer an example. Since many people have read or heard about the links between sunburn and skin cancer, subjects with melanoma may either recall, in greater detail, or exaggerate their sunbathing patterns of the past relative to nonaffected controls. In a case-control study of melanoma in nurses, researchers were fortunate to have collected data related to each subject's ability to tan (a risk for melanoma) as a child both before and after the diagnosis of skin cancer was made.[14] Comparisons were made between cases and controls using both prediagnosis questionnaire results and postdiagnosis results (see Table 3–3). Control subjects' reports were similar for the 2 survey intervals. However, after the diagnosis of melanoma was known, 44% of cases reported poor tanning as a child compared with 26% on the prediagnosis questionnaire.

B. Assessing Subject Bias: Any evidence that researchers have checked on the memory of subjects should be welcome and is notice to the reader that authors are on their toes.

In a case-control study evaluating estrogen therapy given to women to relieve menopausal symptoms and the subsequent risk of developing breast cancer,[15] the authors were aware that the history of drug use given

---

TABLE 3–3

Reported tanning ability among incident cases and controls in a nested case-control study of melanoma, Nurses Health Study cohort, 1976–1984 (in percent)

	Prediagnosis questionnaire		Postdiagnosis questionnaire	
	Incident cases	Controls	Incident cases	Controls
Tanning ability				
No tan to light tan	26	34	44	33
Medium to dark tan	74	66	56	67

Modified, with permission, from Weinstock et al.[14]

by women who had breast cancer might be biased toward the recall of use of estrogens. This was especially likely in view of the substantial controversy the topic has generated in the lay press. The investigators took the additional trouble to review subjects' medical records to document estrogen use as well as to check records from major pharmacies in the community. Thus, 3 estimates of estrogen use were obtained. The researchers were able to show that recall bias did not seem to be playing a role. Estimates of the increased likelihood of breast cancer in high-dosage estrogen users were similar for the 3 data sources.

Alternative sources of data are not always available. Another way of assessing the possible role of recall bias is to note how cases respond to questions that are not related to the outcome. Recall in the study on Reye syndrome that investigators gathered information on ingestion of medications other than aspirin, such as chlorpheniramine and pseudoephedrine. They found no appreciable differences in exposure between cases in the 4 comparison groups (see Table 3–1), evidence that a generalized recollection bias was not operating. Some investigators will even include dummy items—questions they feel are unrelated to melanoma or angina—and see if there is a differential response rate between cases and controls. Case subjects who are exhibiting selective recall may overrespond and identify many items as potentially related to the outcome. So a useful tip for the reader is to take note of how specific the list of associated factors is. If cancer patients recall heavy utilization of 5 or 6 different medications, watch out! If only 1 of a large list of drugs or behaviors has a higher frequency in cases than controls, selective recall is probably less likely.

One might imagine that recall bias could present problems in case-crossover situations. Subjects are asked to report on events that occurred just before an injury or heart attack and similar occurrences in an earlier, less salient time period. Investigators assessing whether heart attacks could be "triggered" by heavy physical exertion needed to learn of patients' level of physical activity in the hour just before the heart attack and compare that to subjects' typical activity patterns.[16] They chose the same time of day 24 hours earlier as a control interval. However, to minimize the bias that might result from focusing subjects on the contrast of the 2 discrete times, researchers imbedded the 2 critical periods in a single "hazard interval" consisting of the entire 26 hours preceding the heart attack. As far as subjects were concerned, the entire "hazard period" was important. Their memories were not prompted to selectively compare the intervals of interest. It turned out that 54 of 1228 subjects had engaged in heavy exertion in the hour immediately preceding the heart attack. This compared with only 9 reporting similar activity levels in the control period the preceding day.

Although not all case-control studies are able to provide evidence that selective recall is not a problem, savvy investigators will at least be cognizant of the importance of this potential bias in their work and report any measures they took to try to master it. The intriguing topic of subject bias has been discussed in several thought-provoking reviews.[17,18]

C. Researcher Bias: When investigators know the identity of case and comparison subjects and which exposures are risks they are seeking, objectivity is put to a strenuous test. It is difficult not to search medical records more thoroughly or question more diligently about exposure to asbestos in cases of fibrotic lung disease or about the consumption of artificial sweeteners among bladder cancer patients. And while such exuberance can be appreciated as an understandable human foible, readers need some assurance that researchers have attempted to guard against potential bias.

In a classic case-control study of smoking and lung cancer published in 1950, the study directors were concerned that interviewers' awareness of which patients had lung cancer might lead them to obtain unequal smoking histories.[19] To test for possible bias, they conducted a substudy in which 100 patients with lung cancer and 186 patients with other chest diseases were interviewed by 2 nonmedical investigators who were unaware of the patients' diagnosis. When distributions of smoking histories for cases and controls in the main study and the substudy were compared, exposure rates were strikingly similar (see Figure 3–1). It appeared, therefore, that interviewer bias was not a problem.

In a study that sought predictive factors in the social environment of patients who had Hodgkin's disease, authors went to elegant lengths to demonstrate that information obtained from controls without cancer was similar to that provided by case patients with Hodgkin's.[20] Interviewers were asked not only to rate the reliability of interviewees but also to record the amount of time spent talking with each subject. The research team was able to report that *information biases* did not appear to be responsible for differences found, since subject reliability was rated as similar for both cases and controls and time spent in the interviews was almost identical, averaging 28.1 and 26.7 minutes for the 2 groups, respectively.

D. Nested Case-Control Studies: Sometimes fortune blesses investigators with a large cohort study that provides useful data from the past and a common population source for cases and controls. The result is a *nested*

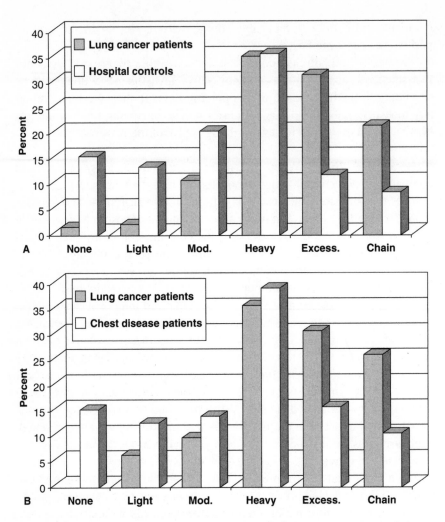

FIGURE 3–1. **A:** Amount of smoking among 605 male patients with lung cancer and 780 general hospital control patients. **B:** Amount of smoking among 100 male patients with lung cancer and 186 male chest disease patients. (Modified, with permission, from Wynder and Graham.[19])

case-control study, or case control within a cohort. Two groups of researchers, both exploring the possible relationship between *Helicobacter pylori* infection and gastric carcinoma, have employed this design with good effect.[21,22] In both instances, large cohorts had been assembled some 20 years earlier. Blood samples were taken and stored. The first cohort consisted of more than 7000 Japanese-American men who enrolled in the

Honolulu Heart Study;[21] the second group was a part of a Kaiser Permanente multiphasic health program.[22] After 20 years, over 100 men from the Honolulu study and 200 from the Kaiser program had been diagnosed with gastric carcinoma. Age-matched controls were selected for each case and antibody titers to *H. pylori* were determined for each pair from the previously collected blood samples. Patients with cancer in both studies demonstrated higher titers, indicating a positive association between prior infection with *H. pylori* and gastric cancer. The nested case-control design created useful information while requiring the analysis of a relatively small number of blood specimens.

A case-control study need not show a difference between exposures among those with and without disease to be of value. A useful "nested" study testing the association between hepatitis B vaccine and subsequent development of multiple sclerosis (MS) was accomplished from within two large cohorts of nurses that make up the Nurses Health Study.[23] These two groups, one of 121,000 female nurses between the ages of 30 and 55 when recruited in 1976, and the other of 116,000 nurses who were in the age group 25–42 when enrollment began in 1989, have provided mountains of useful information through mailed-in questionnaires that are collected every 2 years. Responding to the suggestion that exposure to hepatitis B vaccine may have precipitated the onset of MS, investigators identified 192 nurses who reported the diagnosis. For each case, 5 healthy women were selected as controls, as well as 1 woman with breast cancer. Breast cancer controls were included as a check for recall bias that might occur among patients with the onset of such a serious disease. As previously noted, the use of multiple controls for each case is a technique commonly employed in good case-control methodology. Cases of unusual diseases, such as MS or many cancers, are often available to investigators in limited numbers. Healthy controls are much easier to obtain. Gathering data from 3 or 4 controls for each case improves the investigator's accuracy in estimating the frequency of occurrence of risk factors in the comparison group. It is generally felt that using 3 or 4 controls per case improves accuracy of the study while not sacrificing efficiency.

Evidence of immunization with hepatitis B vaccine within 2 years of the onset of MS was gathered from subject self-reports and checked against immunization records. No increase in exposure to hepatitis B vaccine among cases was found. What was demonstrated was the risk of recall bias. When self-reported dates of vaccination were analyzed, a case of MS had an almost twofold greater likelihood of identifying an immunization within 2 years prior to disease onset. The risk disappeared when only documented immunization dates were used in the analysis. This tendency toward biased recollection was mirrored by the breast cancer control group. They also had higher reports of hepatitis B vaccination within 2 years of the onset of their disease, although there is no known relationship between the vaccine and development of breast cancer.

The nested case-control design is particularly economical when laboratory or other test results are required. Only samples from the subset of cases and controls from the much larger cohort need to be analyzed, a substantial savings in money and effort. The quality and comparability of these data are usually good if they are products of a well-designed follow-up study. The comparability of cases and controls is also high because they come from a common source population and share many social, demographic, and health-risk factors with one another.

Some Last Thoughts on Bias

We have discussed sampling bias, diagnostic bias, reporting bias, and recall bias. Bias can occur any time groups being compared differ systematically in a way that is related to the outcome. Study results may be upset when we fail to recognize important inequalities of information gathering, reporting, sampling, utilization, or observation between groups. Anytime a reader suspects that a group under study goes to doctors more, has more complete records kept, is watched more closely, is questioned more thoroughly, is subjected to more tests, or represents an unusual subgroup of a population, the possibility of bias exists. Patients who are taking potentially hazardous drugs like steroids or estrogens are likely to be observed closely for the occurrence of gastric ulcers or uterine cancer, so these diseases are found at early presymptomatic stages that might go undetected in patients not taking "red-flag" medication. Similarly, patients with diseases that have known risk factors or causes, such as emphysema or bladder cancer, may be questioned in greater detail about these agents than control subjects. *A voluntary response bias* can arise when case subjects who think they have been exposed to a potential carcinogen like arsenic or asbestos return mailed questionnaires at a higher rate than controls. Sackett has listed 35 variations on the bias theme.[24] The names and nuances are of less importance than an understanding of the basic concept.

While readers should be vigilant for the multiple possible sources of bias, it is also well to retain a modicum of perspective. It is not reasonable to dismiss a study as unworthy simply because the possibility for bias exists. Often, when verification of bias (or nonbias) is sought, the information supplied by subjects or data collectors proves quite adequate to the task. Study results may quaver with the threat of biases, but often there is little damage done.

One must also remember that the problems that we have identified may operate in differing directions. Bias may create or accentuate an apparent difference between cases and controls, or it may hide one. A study that finds a strong relationship between coronary artery disease and smoking may include as cases, subjects who are unlikely to have heart disease. But this dilution of cases with noncases will reduce rather than inflate differences between groups. Results would be even more dramatic if our criterion of strict adherence to case definitions were followed. As critical readers, we must assess not only the potential for bias but also the likelihood of its occurrence and actual effect.

SUMMARY

Once a study has been identified as a case-control design, ask the following questions:

1. What kind of population do the cases represent? Are they a valid representation of the disease or outcome in question, or a subset of that population for whom responses are not typical? Have cases been carefully defined to represent a single disease entity or outcome, or are they a mixture of potentially unrelated conditions?

2. How like the case subjects are the controls? Are they drawn from a similar population, differing only in the absence of disease, or are there differences that might bear a relationship to the outcome of the study? If hospital controls are selected, do their diseases bear a relationship to the exposure under study? Are controls likely to overrepresent or underrepresent the exposure status of a general population? If community controls are used, have they been sampled so as to reflect the entire makeup of the community? Have investigators used techniques such as multiple control groups or matching in an effort to improve estimates of exposure among the nondiseased and make controls and cases as comparable as possible?

3. Have data on the exposure in question been accurately obtained from both cases and controls? Are subject or investigator biases creating or masking differences? Do researchers attempt to verify data using multiple sources?

4. Are other biases evident? Do we know more about cases because they have been under closer surveillance, have volunteered more information, or have been subjected to more extensive testing than control subjects?

Passing this critical barrage is a difficult task for a case-control study, but the methods used to conduct studies of this sort are continually improving. A critical look at studies for these common limitations of design may lead to the disquieting conclusion that a number of efforts are not credible. On the other hand, we should feel some joy that investigators are becoming increasingly facile with this challenging methodology and often succeed in providing useful information with maximum efficiency.

REFERENCES

1. Hymes KB et al: Kaposi's sarcoma in homosexual men: A report of eight cases. Lancet 1981;2:598.
2. Illegal fishing [editorial]. Lancet 1981;2:1268.
3. Cassano PA, Koepsell TD, Farwell JR: Risk of febrile seizures in childhood in relation to prenatal maternal cigarette smoking and alcohol intake. Am J Epidemiol 1990;132:462.
4. Klebanoff MA: Invited commentary: The epidemiology of febrile seizures, or the epidemiology of study participation. Am J Epidemiol 1990;132:474.
5. Schlech WF III et al: Risk factors for development of toxic shock syndrome: Association with a tampon brand. JAMA 1982;248:835.
6. Harvey M, Horwitz RI, Feinstein AR: Toxic shock and tampons: Evaluation of the epidemiologic evidence. JAMA 1982;248:840.
7. Hurwitz ES et al: Public Health Service study of Reye's syndrome and medications: Report of the main study. JAMA 1987;257:1905.
8. MacMahon B et al: Coffee and cancer of the pancreas. N Engl J Med 1981;304:630.
9. Silverman DT et al: The prevalence of coffee drinking among hospitalized and population-based control groups. JAMA 1983;249:1877.
10. Oleinick MS et al: Early socialization experiences and intrafamilial environment: A study of psychiatric outpatient and control group children. Arch Gen Psychiatry 1966;15:344.

11. Kernan WN et al: Phenylpropanolamine and the risk of hemorrhagic stroke. N Engl J Med 2000;343:1826.
12. Li G et al: Use of alcohol as a risk factor for bicycling injury. JAMA 2001;285:893.
13. Redelmeier DA, Tibshirani RJ: Association between cellular-telephone calls and motor vehicle collisions. N Engl J Med 1997;336(7):453.
14. Weinstock MA et al: Recall (report) bias and reliability in the retrospective assessment of melanoma risk. Am J Epidemiol 1991;133(3):240.
15. Ross RK et al: A case-control study of menopausal estrogen therapy and breast cancer. JAMA 1980;243:1635.
16. Mittleman MA et al: Triggering of acute myocardial infarction by heavy physical exertion: Protection against triggering by regular exertion. Determinants of Myocardial Infarction Onset Study Investigators. N Engl J Med 1993;329(23):1677.
17. Coughlin SS: Recall bias in epidemiologic studies. J Clin Epidemiol 1990;43:87.
18. Neugebauer R, Ng S: Differential recall as a source of bias in epidemiologic research. J Clin Epidemiol 1990;43:1337.
19. Wynder EL, Graham EA: Tobacco smoking as a possible etiologic factor in bronchiogenic carcinoma: A study of six hundred and eighty-four proved cases. JAMA 1950;143:329.
20. Gutensohn N, Cole P: Childhood social environment and Hodgkin's disease. N Engl J Med 1981;304:135.
21. Nomura A et al: *Helicobacter pylori* and gastric carcinoma among Japanese Americans in Hawaii. N Engl J Med 1991;325:1132.
22. Parsonnet J et al: *Helicobacter pylori* infection and the risk of gastric carcinoma. N Engl J Med 1991;325:1127.
23. Ascherio A et al: Hepatitis B vaccination and the risk of multiple sclerosis. N Engl J Med 2001;344(5):327.
24. Sackett DL: Bias in analytic research. J Chronic Dis 1979;32:51.

CHAPTER FOUR

Study Design: The Cross-Sectional and Follow-up Approaches

Had we but world enough and time,

This cohort study were no crime . . .

But at my back I always hear

Time's winged chariot hurrying near;

—ADAPTED FROM ANDREW MARVELL

From studies that start with subjects who already have an outcome or disease, we will turn to evaluating designs that utilize the cross-sectional and follow-up approaches. As outlined in Chapter 2, these studies tackle the task of providing explanations by assembling groups of subjects that represent either a general, nondiseased population or people who share features we think might predispose them to a particular outcome. Subjects are classified by characteristics such as high cholesterol level, crowded living conditions, or occupational exposure to benzene. Then they are either simultaneously sorted by diseases they already have (for example, heart disease, mental illness, or leukemia) or followed up for a period of time to see what develops.

In the *cross-sectional,* or *prevalence,* approach, it is all done at once, in a single slice of time. A population is chosen for study, a sample of the group is selected, and subjects are poked, probed, and pricked to find out how many have human immunodeficiency virus (HIV) antibody, what the adverse effects from hospital care may be, or how many physicians derive little satisfaction from their medical practices. At the same time, features or risk factors associated with these conditions are elicited. Often the purpose of the exercise is descriptive, to identify the magnitude and details of a health problem. Readers can alert themselves to the likelihood of encountering HIV-positive individuals among prenatal patients or meeting a disgruntled internist in Salt Lake City. On other occasions we are after explanations. Are symptoms of dizziness caused by hypoglycemia? What clinical features best identify patients with bacteremia, or which characteristics of hospitals are associated with poor medical care? Whether the goal is descriptive or explanatory, the same basic strategy applies. The design is schematized in Figure 4–1. Often subjects identified

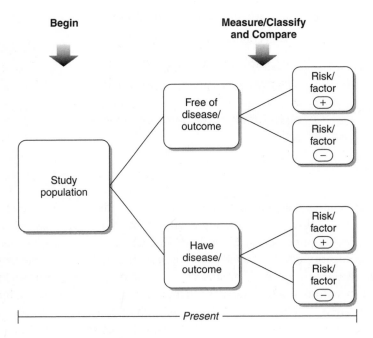

FIGURE 4–1. Cross-sectional study design.

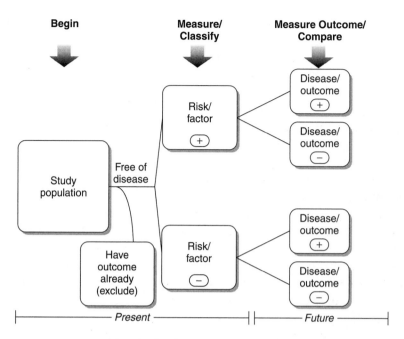

FIGURE 4–2. Follow-up study design.

in these cross-sectional efforts go on to become the cohort or population of interest in a follow-up study. Pregnancies are monitored to find out how many infants become HIV infected, and internists are followed up to see how many leave practice. Figure 4–2 recalls this approach. In this chapter, we will take a closer look at the contributions these study designs can make and learn some critical questions to ask each time one of the strategies is encountered.

CROSS-SECTIONAL DESIGNS

From a quick glance at cross-sectional designs offered in Chapter 2, one might infer that the approach is a country cousin to the more elegant follow-up design. It is true that prevalence studies are often conducted as screening and classification preambles to larger follow-up efforts. Before the incidence of heart disease in a community is studied, the population must be evaluated for current cardiac status and sorted by characteristics such as blood pressure, smoking, and cholesterol level. However, in a number of studies, the cross-sectional design serves as the appetizer, main course, and dessert. The design has considerable flexibility and applicability beyond providing initial classification of patients for subsequent follow-up endeavors. Some of these applications are noted in Table 4–1.

The cross-sectional strategy shares some advantages of the case-control design. It is strong on efficiency. Conclusions are based on information collected at the same time, so investigators are not obliged to wait months or years in the anticipation of an outcome. Everything is done on the spot, often from information that is already at hand. Pharmacy records of antibiotics ordered in a community hospital are searched and usage is detailed according to medical specialty. Patients with juvenile rheumatoid arthritis are tested for histocompatibility antigens and compared by age and symptom patterns. Unfortunately, cross-sectional studies also share frailties with their case-control cousins. High on the list are subject selection and response/participation bias.

TABLE 4–1	
Some uses of the cross-sectional approach	
Use	**Example**
Evaluate a new test or the new application of an old one	Ultrasonography to detect osteoporosis C-reactive protein to predict heart disease risk
Evaluate the predictive capability of clinical features	Relationship of physical examination to bacteremia Accuracy of rectal examination in diagnosing prostate cancer
Identify etiological agents or causative factors	*Salmonella*-induced diarrhea subsequent to church barbecue supper Lactose intolerance as cause of recurrent abdominal pain
Determine the prevalence of a problem	Drug use among health professionals Errors in emergency departments Undertreatment of osteoporosis Enrollment of women in cardiovascular disease trials

Subject Selection

A. Population Selection: The kinds of subjects that find their way into cross-sectional studies can have a major influence on results. It is important to know if the acne patients described as responding favorably to topical treatment with clindamycin are enough like patients we see that comparable therapeutic results may be expected, or that our patients taking birth control pills share features with patients that an article describes as being at increased risk for pulmonary embolism. Sometimes a study offers a view of health risks or outcomes that is accurate for a very special group of patients but that lacks relevance for the practice of the typical clinician. A mismatch is particularly likely when the study population is drawn from a tertiary hospital or referral center. These patients often pass through a complex filter before reaching the meccas. White et al created a model depicting the selection process that takes place before patients arrive at tertiary medical centers.[1] This model has been recently updated, and as seen in Figure 4–3, suggests that only a fraction of potential patients in a

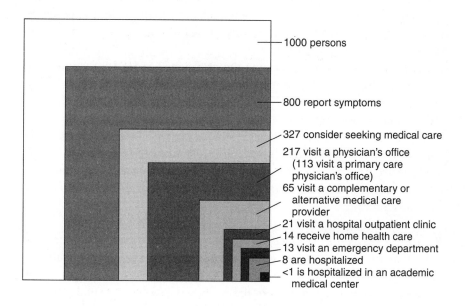

1000 persons

800 report symptoms

327 consider seeking medical care
217 visit a physician's office
   (113 visit a primary care
   physician's office)
65 visit a complementary or
   alternative medical care
   provider
21 visit a hospital outpatient clinic
14 receive home health care
13 visit an emergency department
8 are hospitalized
<1 is hospitalized in an academic
   medical center

FIGURE 4–3. Results of a reanalysis of the monthly prevalence of illness in the community and the roles of various sources of health care. Each box represents a subgroup of the largest box, which comprises 1000 persons. Data are for persons of all ages. (Modified, with permission, from Green et al.[2])

community become subjects for study in a referral center.[2] Those who do are unlikely to be representative of the 999 folks back home. Information gathered on such highly selected patients can be misleading.

An example of population selection at work may be seen from comparing two descriptive studies on the etiology of low back pain. One of these reports comes from the Mayo Clinic,[3] a very special referral center, the other from a family-practice setting.[4] Investigators from each of these sites reviewed the cases of low back pain they had seen over a period of time and described the frequency with which herniated intervertebral disk disease was diagnosed. According to the Mayo Clinic, ruptured disks were responsible for 22% of cases of low back pain; in family practice, only 4.4% of patients with low back pain were suspected of having disk problems, with only 2 of 140 cases reviewed (1.4%) actually confirmed by myelogram and surgically treated. The most likely factor contributing to the varying results is the dissimilarity in the study populations. Most patients who go to Mayo have been to at least one other doctor. Many less important back problems never get referred, so by the time patients reach the clinic, a higher proportion of the pool has more severe disease, such as herniated disks. Physicians in general practice take on all comers and see a greater percentage of less complicated problems. Their experience more accurately reflects the frequency of disk disease in a general population than does the Mayo report.

Surveys designed to determine the prevalence of HIV infection offer another illustration of the importance of population selection. "How many people are infected with HIV?" Estimates vary considerably, depending on the population one surveys.[5] If one samples clinics that treat sexually transmitted diseases, methadone treatment centers, or prisons, the estimate of infected individuals is very different from results obtained from military recruits, Red Cross blood donors, or applicants for marriage licenses. Table 4–2 gives some idea of the variety of estimates obtained from different populations.

B. Sample Selection: Once an author has chosen a population, it is important to find out who within the group becomes a study subject. There is a variety of ways authors can select samples. They may attempt to enroll every eligible subject in the study. That is fine for small populations, but with larger groups, it is not feasible. One approach to dealing with bigger populations is *systematic sampling*, which involves selecting every second or third patient who is available or picking only patients with even numbers as the last digits of their medical records. Another

TABLE 4–2
Seroprevalence of human immunodeficiency virus in different populations

Population	Positives/1000
Homosexual/bisexual men in San Francisco	490
Intravenous drug users in San Francisco	100
Nevada prison inmates	18
Massachusetts newborns	2.0
U.S. military recruits	1.5
Red Cross blood donors	0.2

Modified, with permission, from Centers for Disease Control.[5]

technique is *random sampling*, in which a portion of available patients is chosen by selection of random numbers or drawing from a hat. This assures each member of the population an equal chance of being included in the study. The question that readers must ask is whether the sampling technique employed has guarded against the selection of a biased or unrepresentative sample. Authors may report that patients were selected at random when, in fact, strict randomizing techniques, such as using a random-numbers table or other unbiased procedure, were not used. Used colloquially, the term *random selection* means unplanned or haphazard sampling. It suggests that the authors had no sampling plan in mind but simply took a convenience sample of subjects to enroll in the study. This is not good enough. Very unrepresentative samples of subjects can be obtained when laissez-faire sampling techniques are used.

Let us look at an early study on outpatient blood cultures as an aid to diagnosing the cause of fever in children.[6] This is a good example of a cross-sectional design that seeks evidence for the utility of the application of a test (blood cultures) to clarify a clinical problem (fever of unknown origin). All febrile children attending a walk-in clinic during a 3-month period were eligible for study. Blood cultures were obtained from these children to ascertain the prevalence of bacteremia, and subjects were simultaneously cross-classified by characteristics such as degree of fever, age, and white blood cell count to augment the clinician's predictive power (see Table 4–3).

TABLE 4–3	
Factors associated with bacteremia in febrile children	
Factor	**Percent of patients with positive blood cultures**
Fever	
<38.9°C	0.9
38.9-39.9°C	6.6
40.0°C or higher	8.0
Age	
<12 months	6.7
13-24 months	4.6
25 months or older	2.7
White blood cell count	
<10,000/mm³	1.1
10,000-19,900/mm³	6.1
≥20,000/mm³	11.6

Modified, with permission, from McGowan et al.[6]

The authors do well in clearly defining fever as a "rectal temperature of 38.3°C or higher or an oral temperature of 37.8°C or higher," but they report as their sampling technique only that "physicians of the pediatric service were requested to obtain a blood culture from febrile patients." It turns out that during the 3-month study period, 2059 children who met the fever criteria visited the clinic. Of these, only 415, or 20%, actually had blood cultures obtained. In other words, only one-fifth of eligible patients were included. With no more information than we have at hand regarding the sampling procedure, can we assume that the children included represent the entire population in an unbiased fashion? Probably not. Children on whom blood cultures were done are likely to have been kids who worried physicians because they appeared to have a toxic condition; that is, they were suspected of having a bacterial infection such as pneumonia or meningitis. Youngsters who appeared to have benign febrile illnesses, such as roseola or viral gastroenteritis, would be less promising candidates for culture. Any estimate of the frequency of bacteremia in this selected sample is probably an overestimate of the likelihood of positive blood cultures among the broader population of febrile children. The results may give us an idea of how often bacteria can be isolated from the blood of very sick youngsters, but without a clear description of the selection that went on, we have no way of generalizing the data. Had the authors provided us with comparative information about the clinical condition of the patients sampled and those excluded, the data they provide might be more useful.

The question of HIV prevalence provides another example of sampling problems. To estimate the occurrence of HIV infection among university students in the United States, blood samples from 19 universities across the country were collected and tested for antibodies to HIV.[7] Of almost 17,000 specimens collected, 30, or 0.2%, had detectable HIV antibodies. This rate of 1 positive for 500 students tested was acknowledged to be lower than rates found among high-risk groups, but it was greater than the prevalence of 0.15% found in civilian applicants for military service.[5] The popular press reported on the study findings and extrapolated results to estimate that 25,000 college students across the nation may be infected with HIV.

However, the sampling techniques used in this project raise serious questions about the validity of such claims. In an attempt to maintain confidentiality, the serosurvey was conducted not on a random sample of students at the 19 universities but on a *convenience sample* of blood specimens that were collected at university health centers in the course of clinical care. While such a procedure may be desirable from the privacy perspective, it creates an unsatisfactory sample. We know nothing about the study participants except that they visited the health services and had conditions that clinicians felt required a blood test. It is likely that some made clinic visits related to sexually transmitted diseases, and some may have been concerned that they had been exposed to HIV. Students who visit health centers and have blood taken are not representative of the general student body.

Response/Participation Bias

Even when a population is carefully chosen and samples are selected to provide accurate estimates of that population, studies can suffer if subjects do not cooperate. Lack of participation may occur for a host of reasons. Subjects may have moved or cannot be contacted, they may be too ill to participate or even have died, or they may decline participation for a variety of personal reasons. The chief concern is, of course, that people who agree to answer questions and submit to blood tests differ from those who do not. If systematic dissimilarities between participants and nonparticipants are related to the outcomes we are attempting to measure, results may be distorted.

At the start of a follow-up study of coronary heart disease and stroke among men of Japanese ancestry who were living in Honolulu, 73% of approximately 11,000 eligible men agreed to participate and submit to a baseline physical examination.[8] That left almost 3000 nonparticipants. Fortunately, investigators had distributed a mailed questionnaire requesting information on certain biological and lifestyle characteristics. Because this had been returned by 60% of men who subsequently declined participation in the larger study, certain features of participants and nonparticipants could be compared. It was discovered that the two groups differed significantly in several important respects. Participants were more likely to be married, to have a high school education, to have been previously hospitalized, and to be nonsmokers. When mortality figures for the two groups were assessed 14 years later, participants, with their lower risk profiles, had significantly lower mortality than nonparticipants.

The case-control study of bicycle injury and alcohol use discussed in Chapter 3 offers several opportunities for participation bias.[9] Control subjects were bicyclists who were approached by interviewers and asked to volunteer for an alcohol breath test. The authors note that cyclists who have been drinking might be less likely to stop or to participate in the study. The frequency of alcohol use among controls thus would be underestimated. Similarly, not all injured cases identified in the trauma registry had blood alcohol concentrations recorded. If obtaining a blood alcohol level was related to the clinician's suspicion that an individual was intoxicated, blood tests might have been omitted on people doctors thought were sober, and estimates of the frequency of drinking among cases then would be spuriously high.

Unfortunately, because they are nonresponders, there is often lack of information on nonparticipants that can be used to assess such bias. Investigators should share what information they have on the comparability of respondents and nonrespondents. Supplying readers with the response or participation rate is a minimum requirement. How high the rate should be to be considered acceptable is a matter of debate. Rates in excess of 80% are considered very good by most, and those below 40% as suspicious. Obviously, even relatively small groups of nonresponders may differ in important ways from their parent populations, as the Honolulu Heart Study example illustrates. Any sort of demographic or risk-factor information that authors can supply to clarify the situation is helpful. Details as to why folks declined participation can also be of use.

Time-Order Relationships

Cross-sectional studies fall prey to a chicken-and-egg dilemma. Since information related to a subject's outcome is collected at the same time as data on the possible causative or predictive factor, it is not always clear which comes first. Does the attribute or characteristic really lead to the effect or disease, or does the outcome in some way predispose people to acquire factors or characteristics that appear to be predictive?

Researchers investigating the relationship between obesity and "nonexercise activity" of daily routines examined the habitual body postures of 20 self-proclaimed "couch potatoes" over the course of 10 days.[10] Ten of the subjects were lean and 10 were mildly obese. Sophisticated measuring devices enabled the collection of about 25 million data points on movement and posture for each volunteer. Findings revealed that obese subjects spent 164 minutes longer each day sitting than lean participants, and the latter group 154 minutes longer standing upright. The amount of time spent sleeping was similar. The difference in the habitual activity patterns of the two groups translated into an expenditure of 352 calories per day, an explanation for the excess weight among the heavier couch potatoes.

However, the researchers recognized that the lower daily activity may not be responsible for increased weight. Rather, being overweight leads to less activity. To test whether differences in habitual posture were a *cause* rather than a *consequence* of obesity, they intervened in their otherwise observational effort. Obese volunteers underwent a weight loss program (losing an average of 8 kg over 8 weeks) and lean subjects were overfed during the same time interval (gaining an average of 4 kg). Posture measurements were repeated and the findings were unchanged. Notwithstanding the rather brief duration of the change in weight, the investigators suggest that differences in posture lead to obesity and appear to be biologically determined.

Self-Reported Information

Observational studies are susceptible to inaccuracies in the information that is acquired for either exposures (as discussed in Chapter 3) or outcomes. Data on health events are often most easily obtained directly from study subjects themselves but even when the information sought has high salience there can be problems. When investigators from New Zealand were collecting data for a large World Health Organization study on heart disease, they gathered information directly from participants on recent hospitalizations.[11] The availability of New Zealand's computerized national database with records on all hospitalizations in the country gave the researchers an opportunity to verify these subject reports. They were far from perfect. Of the 524 participants studied, very few indicated a hospitalization that was not documented in the national database. But when it came to reporting admissions, only 58% recalled all those the computer had on record. Sixteen percent recalled none of their documented admissions. This is not happy news. Often external validation of self-reports is not feasible, but when possible, it is an activity that lends credibility to results.

Variations on the Theme

1. Sequential Cross-Sectional Studies: Cross-sectional studies may be repeated at several time intervals, then combined to depict trends that alert us to the progress we are making on solving health problems or the need to increase our efforts. Large sequential cross-sectional surveys show us that rates of smoking are declining in the population, seat-belt use is reluctantly increasing, and measles immunization rates have fallen to embarrassing levels. This approach, also called a *time-series*, can provide useful information. And for large, well-constructed surveys like many conducted by the National Center for Health Statistics, the information is quite dependable. However, trends are built upon repeated cross-sectional studies, which assume that representative sampling of the same parent population takes place. If the composition of the reference population changes over time, if sampling is altered, or if patterns of response change, apparent trends in seat-belt use may be due to quirks of method rather than health behavior. The HIV/AIDS literature again provides instruction.

Investigators from the New York State Department of Health provided seropositivity information for a number of New York State HIV testing sites over several years.[12] Data on the numbers of individuals tested and the percentage with positive tests over 4 sequential time periods are shown in Table 4–4.

If one were presented with only the data from the top rows of the table, the trend would appear to be encouraging. The percentage of patients with positive results falls from 14.5 to 4.2%, while the number of

TABLE 4–4				
Serologic testing for human immunodeficiency virus over 4 periods of time				
	1/86–6/86	**7/86–12/86**	**1/87–6/87**	**7/87–12/87**
Number tested	2127	2374	4989	7602
Percent positive	14.5	13.6	5.7	4.2
% male	72.5	66.4	57.8	56.3
% symptomatic	17.7	16.4	8.0	8.0
% IV drug user	15.0	14.9	10.9	10.8
% homo/bisexual	42.9	39.7	26.1	24.6

Modified, with permission, from Grabau and Morse.[12]

patients tested grows. One might conclude that infection with HIV is on the wane and the epidemic in decline. However, the authors provide additional information that dampens any such optimism. When questionnaire data obtained from those tested are added to the table, substantial changes in the composition of the groups studied in the sequential periods are evident. The proportion of individuals with high-risk behaviors for HIV infection or who were experiencing symptoms fell over time. Greater numbers of lower-risk individuals sought testing. The fall in HIV seroprevalence cannot be attributed to declining rates of infection without accounting for the dramatic changes in the population undergoing testing.

2. Ecologic Studies: A research approach that is often accorded its own place among methods taxonomies is the *ecologic* design. Contrary to expectations, these are not studies bent on preserving the natural habitat. The design is actually cross-sectional in structure. Its distinction lies in the type of data that is collected. Up to this point, we have assumed that information on risks or exposures and diseases or outcomes comes from individuals. We expect that alcohol levels are measured on those who are in the bicycle crashes, and vaccination records are reviewed for patients with multiple sclerosis. Ecologic studies use data from groups. Comparisons are made, for example, between national rates of heart disease among countries where typical diets are low or high in fat. Cancer rates are checked in farming counties and correlated with pesticide sales. Rates of motorcycle collision fatalities are compared among states with and without helmet laws.

The ecological approach has been widely used in studies relating air pollution to adverse health events. In one example, 5 major outdoor air pollutants were measured on a daily basis in 20 metropolitan areas around the United States.[13] Air samplers were placed at strategic points in each city to gather information on particulate matter, ozone, sulfur dioxide, carbon monoxide, and nitrogen dioxide. Twenty-four-hour averages of these pollutants were then compared with the mean number of deaths that occur each day in the particular urban location. Researchers found a clear relationship between concentrations of fine particulates in the environment and mortality. When they homed in on deaths from cardiovascular and respiratory diseases, those most likely to be exacerbated or caused by pollution, their hypothesis was further supported.

Geographic regions with different environmental exposures provide useful grist for ecologic studies. But any groups where there are notable differences in potential risk behaviors may be suitable subjects for the design. When researchers compared the mortality experience of medical graduates from Loma Linda University with that of alums from nearby University of Southern California, they found that the Loma Linda physicians' death rate was only three-quarters that of their Southern California colleagues.[14] The explanation proposed by this study is Loma Linda's strong affiliation with the Seventh-Day Adventist Church, a group that subscribes to vegetarian diets and avoids the use of tobacco and alcohol.

Ecologic data can also be used in a time-series approach. Data on per capita cigarette consumption and mortality from heart disease in the state of California were tracked over a period of time in which the state enacted a tobacco control program.[15] Sequential cross-sectional surveys compared the statewide heart disease death rate each year with the same year's data on per capita cigarette sales. Cigarette consumption in California falls more rapidly than the rest of the United States in the years the tobacco program is in force. Heart disease deaths decline in parallel to the reduced consumption. When, several years after initiation, the tobacco program sustains serious cutbacks, the reductions in cigarette sales and heart disease mortality level off. Again, there are no individual data. We do not know if those who die of heart disease are cigarette smokers or not. We have only average mortality figures and annual cigarette sales reports.

This all may seem a rather crude approximation of exposure. Huge lumps of aggregate data take the place of precise estimates of individual exposures. Most texts on the subject are quick to point out this failing. The individuals within the groups being assessed may not, in fact, be the ones who are exposed to the risk factor. It is known as *ecologic fallacy*.

Many say that the ecologic approach is only useful for hypothesis generating and rarely supplies definitive information, but there are virtues in the method. It is highly efficient and economical. The expense and time required to assemble large groups of subjects and conduct detailed measurements on their habits is replaced by simply gathering data that are already available. The ecologic approach can address problems that would be difficult to study at the individual level. Mortality related to air pollution is a case in point. It is hard to imagine attaching an air sampler to each of the thousands of individuals who would be needed to estimate individual respiratory exposures. Measurements on groups may also be appropriate when one is trying to assess the impact of a broadly based health initiative, such as a law. We may not have individual data on whether particular individuals who are injured in motorcycle accidents after passage of a helmet law were wearing helmets, but if fatalities decline noticeably, we have some evidence that the legislation may be having an effect.

A further problem that hinders firm conclusions from ecologic studies comes from knowledge that factors other than those being measured may be responsible for the outcomes. A massive movement toward low-fat diets and more exercise might have occurred in California at the same time the tobacco control program was in full swing. Changes in diet and physical activity rather than in smoking might have been responsible for the drop in deaths from heart disease.

FOLLOW-UP STUDIES

The *follow-up,* or *cohort,* design is generally considered to be the crème de la crème of observational methodologies. It is unencumbered by many of the problems that beset the case-control and cross-sectional approaches. Since data are gathered prospectively rather than from rooting through records of the past, they may be collected in a comprehensive and uniform fashion. There is no need to worry about whether height and weight were recorded in the chart or whether blood pressure was accurately measured. Investigators can set up the rules before they begin. Nor is recall bias a problem, since patients are not being asked to recall events of the past but will be followed into the future to see which outcomes develop. Time-order relationships are also made clear, because patients are classified by characteristics before the disease or outcome becomes manifest.

It is all much tidier, there is much more control over the quality of the data, and there is greater clarity in the sequence of events. Had we, as Andrew Marvell suggests, no constraints of resources and unlimited time, it would be the ideal strategy. Unfortunately, substantial costs are likely to be incurred in following large populations, and "time's winged chariot" does, in fact, press us.

Follow-up studies are also not without their methodological weak points. In addition to that persistent plague, population selection, there are 3 other afflictions that we have not examined thus far: loss to follow-up, changes in subject characteristics, and surveillance bias.

Selection

Follow-up designs are susceptible to selection problems. An elegant illustration comes from the literature on febrile convulsions in children. In a typical case, a toddler 1–2 years of age will be bundled to the emergency room by frantic parents. The child seemed fine, they report, until he suddenly fell to the floor, eyes rolled back, in a generalized convulsion. The seizure lasted for only a few minutes, and not until the aftermath did the parents realize the child was febrile to 104°F. This is a horrifying experience for parents. When the initial anxiety abates, their most immediate concerns are, "Will it happen again?" and "Does this mean my child has epilepsy?" These are good questions—just the kind that require a good follow-up study to answer. The answers, however, are very much dependent on the kind of population whose natural history is assessed. A study from Edinburgh, for example, followed up 200 children admitted to a teaching hospital with the diagnosis of febrile convulsion.[16] The researchers found that almost 17% of these children had subsequent nonfebrile recurrences, which is quite a large number. However, if the response to parents about epilepsy is based on a Greek study, febrile seizure patients will have a 65% chance of having later nonfebrile seizures.[17] For those who find this prospect much too distressing, Nelson and Ellenberg give an overall risk of nonfebrile recurrences of only 3%.[18] That's certainly more encouraging! With such a wide variety of results, all coming from reputable journals, how do we know whom to believe?

In fact, all these studies may be right. They may all accurately portray the risk of recurrent seizures for the particular population they are observing. Readers must decide how the groups of patients reported compare with those they will be seeing. In this particular situation, the Scottish study reports on children who were hospitalized at a large medical center, the Greek study describes patients referred to a special developmental evaluation center, and Nelson's patients come from a cohort of 54,000 newborn infants from 11 U.S. cities who were followed up for some years to detect neurological abnormalities. Ethnic differences notwithstanding, the broad population sample best reflects the kind of patients most doctors encounter and suggests that for most children who experience febrile convulsions, the risk of subsequent, nonfebrile attacks is small.

To confirm their impression that sample selection plays an important role in the results one finds, Ellenberg and Nelson made some further comparisons.[19] They reviewed 26 published articles that estimated the likelihood of nonfebrile seizures for children with febrile fits and classified findings by 2 categories of study populations. One group was composed of clinic-based studies—those that followed up patients who came from hospital clinics or specialty referral units. The other group contained population-based studies—where a clearly defined general population was used. The comparative rates of recurrence are depicted in Figure 4–4.

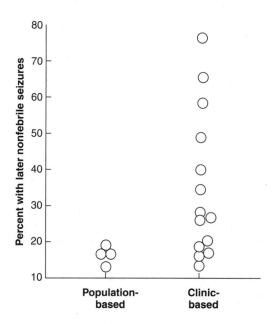

FIGURE 4–4. Percentage of children who experienced nonfebrile seizures after one or more febrile seizures in population-based (**left**) and clinic-based (**right**) studies. (Modified, with permission, from Ellenberg and Nelson.[19])

Estimates for clinic-based studies are highly variable, ranging up to 75%; figures derived from population-based studies are much lower and remarkably consistent at about 3%.

Every study will have its own population of subjects, and each will have limits of generalizability. Readers must decide how closely subjects described in the study mirror patients they will be treating. Good authors will help in this task. Readers have a right to expect a reasonable amount of information about patients described in any study. What are their demographic characteristics? Where do they come from? Have they been referred from other medical care facilities, or have they come on their own? What is the reputation of the facility where the patients were gathered? Is it known to attract certain kinds of patients with certain kinds of illnesses? Is it a specialty clinic? Only armed with this information can the reader address the problem of external validity or generalizability. If our patients are very unlike those being described in the study, we may be justified in feeling some reluctance to embrace the author's conclusions.

Loss to Follow-up

No matter how carefully one's sample is chosen, no matter how elegantly representative of the population, if subjects are lost to follow-up, we are in trouble. The biggest single problem of follow-up-design investigations is the loss of valuable information through attrition. Subjects change addresses, fail to respond to questionnaires, decide they no longer wish to participate, or just plain cannot be located. Dropouts are unfortunate, not simply because they reduce the numbers of subjects observed but also because the reasons subjects become lost to follow-up may be related to the outcomes under study. That adds another potential source of bias.

An illustration comes from the report of a study on the likelihood that women who lose babies will become depressed during the 6-month postpartum period.[20] Study subjects included women who had had a stillborn infant or whose baby died in the first 7 days of life. A complete sample of mothers who lost babies was taken for a year in an entire English county. For each of these, a comparison subject was chosen from all the mothers residing in the same locale who had had live births in that year. The authors matched the cases and controls by place and time of delivery. It is worth recalling here that while the authors speak of these comparison mothers as controls and refer to perinatal death subjects as cases, they are not utilizing a case-control design. The action of the study is forward, and perinatal death is not the outcome but a potential risk factor for postpartum depression. The authors are forced to sample from the total pool of comparison patients, since to have included all live births would have created an extremely large cohort.

Questionnaires were given out at 2 days, 6 days, 6 weeks, and 6 months postpartum, asking women to report on symptoms related to depression. When returned questionnaires were tallied and evaluated for the presence of depressive symptomatology, a rather surprising finding emerged. "At 6 months, postpartum depression was just as common in women aged under 24 whose babies had survived as in women of the same age whose babies had died." This revelation is certainly contrary to what one would expect. Unfortunately, diligent as the authors were in their attempts to keep track of the women they enrolled in the study, not everyone responded to the questionnaire. And there is reason to believe that this loss to follow-up was biased. The authors note that "compared with the control group, fewer of the women whose babies had died responded to the six-month questionnaire." It also happens that in both groups the nonresponse rate was "more than twice as high" for women whose day 2 depression scores were high than for those whose rating indicated no depression. This information has some sticky implications. If women failed to respond to questionnaires because they were depressed, the unexpectedly low rate of postpartum depression among women who lost babies is an artifact of biased follow-up. These women are depressed— so depressed they are not up to completing and returning a depression inventory.

Subject loss is the bane of the follow-up study. A questionnaire is sent to patients asking them to report their satisfaction with a recent visit to the clinic. Only 50% respond. Are those who do not respond failing to do so because they are angry and dissatisfied, or because they are pleased with the service and have no complaints? A study is designed to follow up respiratory function of workers who have occupational exposure to cotton dust. A substantial number of workers cannot be located 10 years later, when it is time to evaluate their pulmonary status. Is there anything special about the group that cannot be found? Have they all changed jobs because of respiratory incapacity? Have they moved to Arizona so that they can breathe? The possibility that attrition in studies is due to the factors being explored is substantial.

There are several ways that investigators can deal with the follow-up problem. Canny readers should check behind the author to see if this homework has been performed.

1. Have the investigators made every effort to track down lost subjects? Repeated mailings, telephone contacts, or home visits give evidence that investigators have been diligent in their efforts to locate wayward subjects and suggest concern about attrition. The authors of the report on perinatal death and depression get positive marks for their effort.[20] Second mailings were sent to all nonresponders to the first letter, and health visitors were sent to homes of those who failed to respond to the second mailing. Losses still occurred.

2. Do authors report the rate of follow-up loss and explore the possibility of biased attrition? Recognizing that some loss is inevitable, authors should detail the extent of the problem and offer information on characteristics of the nonrespondents. Authors should be able to provide demographic features, such as age, sex, and some initial classifying information like responses to the first depression scale. The more information indicating that the lost sheep are similar to those in the fold, the more comfortable we may feel that an important attrition bias is not influencing results. Any follow-up study that fails to offer information on losses should be viewed with skepticism.

3. Another technique for characterizing nonrespondents or dropouts is to spend some additional effort to contact a representative sample of this total group. This may be a difficult task, since initial efforts at contact have been unsuccessful; but the effort expended in attacking a small sample may reward the investigator with important information about the characteristics of these lost subjects.

Change in Habits

Although the follow-up design appears to avoid the messy business of relying on the memories of subjects to catalog habits and exposures of the past, other snares await the best-laid plans. Subjects can change their habits. Smokers quit smoking, the inactive take up jogging, and dieters stop using saccharine. When investigators rely on initial categorizations of smoking activity and use of artificial sweeteners, they may find themselves misclassifying subjects. People thought to be at high risk may alter their lifestyle or reduce their exposure to a drug or environmental contaminant. Those who are thought to be at low risk may begin snacking on potato chips or start work as asbestos removers. If only small numbers of subjects change their roles in an unselected way, there is not much problem; if many people switch, it can be trouble. In the time it takes to follow up on the natural history of a group of people, many uncontrolled outside events can occur. A community health education campaign may induce subjects to stop smoking, or a national fad such as jogging may overtake even the most sedentary of the citizenry. Patients may read in the newspaper about the dangerous side effects of a drug they have been taking and decide to discontinue the medication. There is not a great deal investigators can do to control this phenomenon, but they can periodically reexamine subjects and update classifications. The large Nurses Health Study resurveys their subjects every 2 years. Readers should look for evidence that authors are alert to the issue and reexamine their cohort to see whether habits or exposures have changed.

Surveillance Bias

Another bias in follow-up studies can occur if there is unequal surveillance of subjects being compared. This problem is shared by all the observational designs and occurs any time one group of subjects gets scrutinized or examined more closely than others. A case in point is a follow-up study that describes antecedents of child abuse and neglect among premature infants.[21] Investigators collected extensive information on 255 families who had infants admitted to the newborn intensive care unit of a university medical center. A "psychosocial risk inventory" was created to help identify children who might be subsequent victims of child abuse. Included in the inventory was information such as adequacy of child spacing, social isolation, major life stress, adequacy of child-care arrangements, and financial status. Each family was scored and categorized as being at high or low psychosocial risk. The authors found that after a follow-up period of 6–19 months, 10 of 41 infants (24%) assigned to the high-risk group were reported to be abused or neglected, compared with none of the infants categorized as being at low psychosocial risk.

That is an impressive difference and suggests that the psychosocial scoring system has great utility. Unfortunately, a misstep in design opens the way for significant surveillance bias. Infants who were classified as high risk on the basis of their inventory scores were identified to social service agencies at the time of discharge from the hospital. While this may have been desirable practice from the viewpoint of supporting families in need of help, it seriously interferes with the ability to give an unbiased assessment of the value of the scoring system. Identifying the infants as at high risk for abuse also puts them at high risk of close surveillance and at high risk for being reported for abuse and neglect. It is like examining one group of histological specimens under low-power scan and another group under oil immersion. The closer you look, the more you find. Reading that evidence of neglect included "leaving infants unattended at home, failing to comply with routine immunizations, and failing to provide adequate nutrition" suggests that differential surveillance is contributing to the findings. Low-risk kids are probably also being left unattended—but no one is watching.

SUMMARY

Having come across a study design you identify as being a cross-sectional or follow-up approach, consider the following questions:

1. How is the study population selected? Do subjects come from a referral center, a general medical practice, or the community at large? Are there special features or characteristics of patients that would select them for membership in this particular population? Are they older, sicker, or richer, or do they have more severe manifestations of a given disease? Have they already come through selective filters in the medical system? Do the authors provide sufficient information for you to identify the population and judge its similarity to your own?

2. Are procedures for sampling within this population clearly defined? Can you tell exactly how individual subjects were picked? Were they chosen in a manner that avoids selection bias? Do authors provide evidence that subjects who are eligible but not included in the study are similar to those that have been selected? Do authors acknowledge the potential for selection bias and give evidence of safeguards used to avoid it or demonstrate that the problem has not affected results?

3. Is participation or subject response bias occurring? Have authors included the participation or response rate in their results? Has an attempt been made to characterize nonparticipants? Are they

angrier, happier, or less health conscious than those who agreed to the study? Are differences in these characteristics related to outcomes and likely to bias results?

4. When a cross-sectional approach is utilized, are time-order relationships clear? If subjects are simultaneously classified by behaviors or potentially causative characteristics and the effects or outcomes, is cause and effect implied when the sequence of events is not clear? Is it likely that the characteristic really leads to the outcome, or could people who have certain diseases secondarily acquire characteristics that appear causative?

5. If a follow-up design is utilized, is there loss to follow-up? Are authors careful to detail the methods used to follow up on subjects and provide information about subjects who stay? Are these nonrespondents or dropouts likely to bias results? Are reasons for attrition likely to be related to outcomes under study? Did subjects fail to answer because they were depressed or had left town because they could not breathe?

6. Did subjects change habits or exposures during the course of study? Have those believed to be at high risk initially changed their status by altering lifestyle, occupation, or drug intake? Do authors periodically reexamine their cohorts to see if habits have changed?

7. Is surveillance bias occurring? Are the groups being compared being observed with equal intensity? Or is high-powered scrutiny being applied to certain subjects, which may bias results?

REFERENCES

1. White KL, Williams TF, Greenberg BG: The ecology of medical care. N Engl J Med 1961;265:885.
2. Green L et al: The ecology of medical care revisited. N Engl J Med 2001;344(26):2012.
3. Ghormley RK: An etiology study of backache and sciatic pain. Proceedings of the Staff Meetings of the Mayo Clinic 1951;26:457.
4. Barton JE et al: Low back pain in the primary care setting. J Fam Pract 1976;3:363.
5. Centers for Disease Control: Human immunodeficiency virus infection in the United States: A review of current knowledge. MMWR 1987;36(suppl S6):22.

6. McGowan JE Jr et al: Bacteremia in febrile children seen in a "walk-in" pediatric clinic. N Engl J Med 1973;288:1309.
7. Gayle HD et al: Prevalence of the human immunodeficiency virus among university students. N Engl J Med 1990;323:1538.
8. Benfante R et al: Response bias in the Honolulu heart program. Am J Epidemiol 1989;130:1088.
9. Li G, Smialck JE, Soderstrom CA: Use of alcohol as a risk factor for bicycling injury. JAMA 2001;285:893.
10. Levine JA et al: Individual variation in posture allocation: Possible role in human obesity. Science 2005;307:584.
11. Norrish A et al: Validity of self-reported hospital admission in a prospective study. Am J Epidemiol 1994;140(10):938.
12. Grabau JC, Morse DL: Seropositivity for HIV at alternate sites. JAMA 1988;260:3128.
13. Samet JM et al: The National Morbidity, Mortality, and Air Pollution Study. Part I: Methods and methodologic issues. Res Rep Health Eff Inst 2000(94 Pt 1):5; discussion 75.
14. Ullmann D et al: Cause-specific mortality among physicians with differing life-styles. JAMA 1991;265(18):2352.
15. Fichtenberg CM, Glantz SA: Association of the California Tobacco Control Program with declines in cigarette consumption and mortality from heart disease. N Engl J Med 2000;343(24):1772.
16. Wallace SJ: Spontaneous fits after convulsions with fever. Arch Dis Child 1977;52:192.
17. Gregoriades AD: A medical and social survey of 231 children with seizures. Epilepsia 1972;13:13.
18. Nelson KB, Ellenberg JH: Predictors of epilepsy in children who have experienced febrile seizures. N Engl J Med 1976;295:1029.
19. Ellenberg JH, Nelson KB: Sample selection and the natural history of disease: Studies of febrile seizures. JAMA 1980;243:1337.
20. Clarke M, Williams AJ: Depression in women after perinatal death. Lancet 1979;1:916.
21. Hunter RS et al: Antecedents of child abuse and neglect in premature infants: A prospective study in a newborn intensive care unit. Pediatrics 1978;61:629.

CHAPTER FIVE

Study Design: The Experimental Approach

*I took 12 patients in the scurvy . . . two of these were ordered each
a quart of cider . . . Two others took 25 gutts of elixer vitriol . . .
two took two spoonfuls of vinegar . . . two were put under a
course of sea-water . . . two others had each two oranges and one
lemon . . . two took the bigness of a nutmeg three-times-a-day. . . .*

JAMES LIND, *A TREATISE OF THE SCURVY*

Let us now sing the praises of the controlled trial! Although its ancestry
certainly dates back to the eighteenth century, when James Lind fed
12 British sailors everything from seawater and vinegar to oranges (not limes)
in an attempt to treat scurvy, wide acceptance of the experimental strategy is
a relatively recent occurrence. The British trials on the chemotherapy of
tuberculosis performed in the late 1940s by many accounts mark the birth of
the modern fascination with the controlled trial. The controlled trial represents the only study design available for clinical researchers that approximates the laboratory experiment. Most noted as a recipe for comparing drug
therapies, the technique has evolved into a tool for evaluating a wide variety
of clinical problems. Examples include the use of the controlled trial to compare methods of childbirth, to study medical versus surgical treatment of

coronary artery disease, and to assess relaxation and meditation as a means of reducing high blood pressure. The scope of the design has broadened to include what are, strictly speaking, nonclinical areas of concern, such as health services, education, and health administration. Trials have been created to evaluate the efficacy of nurse practitioners compared with physicians and to judge the effectiveness of campaigns promoting the use of seat belts.

Certainly, after dealing with the frustrating biases of the roundabout strategies of observational studies, the controlled trial presents a refreshing, direct approach. The many difficulties of studying populations in their free-living state appear to be obviated by the planned comparisons of drugs or surgical techniques, health education programs, or administrative innovations that are possible with the controlled trial design. Life for researchers is much simpler when they have some control over interventions. Nevertheless, even controlled trials have some associated tribulations that medical readers must know about. The need to have high-quality information on interventions from trials has spawned groups that have produced useful information on assessing the methodology. One such group, known as CONSORT (Consolidated Standards

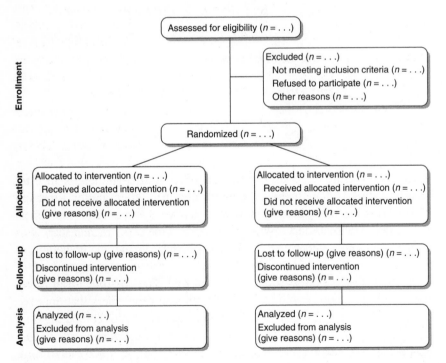

FIGURE 5–1. Flow diagram of subject progress through the phases of a randomized trial. (Modified, with permission, from Moher et al.[1])

for Reporting of Trials), has published guidelines detailing the elements that should be included in reports of randomized trials.[1] They have created a flow diagram that is a particularly useful guide for assessing articles that report trial results. It is reproduced as Figure 5–1 and will serve as a framework for our discussion.

We will look at 4 major areas of methodological concern. The first of these has to do with *enrollment,* how people get into the study. Next, we will address *allocation,* ways subjects are chosen and assigned to their particular study groups. We will examine *follow-up* and expand on several issues raised in Chapter 4. Finally, we will explore some features of *analysis* that are special to the controlled trial. It will be a plateful.

ENROLLMENT: WHO GETS IN

The Study Population & Entry Criteria

As we have seen before, the people an investigator chooses to study make a big difference. Results obtained from hospital settings do not necessarily translate to primary care clinics or general populations. Experimental studies are also susceptible to selection problems. However, there are some added twists—both the populations selected for study and those who are actually enrolled in the trials need to be considered.

When investigators from Boston wished to test aspirin as a primary preventative for myocardial infarction, they elected to use a special group of subjects: physicians.[2] Doctors, they reasoned, make excellent subjects in several respects. Physicians are well informed about the risks and benefits of such a trial, they are accurate personal historians, and they are easier to track for follow-up than many people in the general population. The downside is that doctors are hardly a representative slice of people in the United States. In the Physicians' Health Study (PHS),[*] subjects were

---

[*]The Physicians' Health Study was actually designed to test *two* interventions simultaneously, aspirin for heart attack and beta-carotene for cancer. Because the interventions were aimed at two unrelated health problems and the mechanisms of effect are presumed to operate independently, a "factorial design" was employed. Subjects were allocated first to treatment with aspirin or placebo, then to beta-carotene or placebo. Some folks get aspirin and beta-carotene, some get only one of the two, and some have only placebo tablets in their pill packets. It is an efficient way to answer two questions for the price of one.

all male, were relatively young (40% were younger than 50), and had better health habits than most citizens. So the question must be asked, "Are results that accrue from these willing, healthy, male doctors applicable to the general population of people who are hoping to avoid heart attack?" Will findings apply to women, to men with less socioeconomic privilege, or to those who pay less attention to their health? It may be that, as the investigators argue, "there seems little reason to suspect that the biological effects of aspirin would be materially different in other populations with comparable or higher risk of cardiovascular disease."[2] But one worries. Even the investigators were somewhat unsettled by the finding that, "while 733 cardiovascular deaths were expected based on mortality rates from the general population of US males of that age, only 88 were observed."[2] That is a pretty healthy bunch of doctors.

Once the general study population has been chosen, a second kind of selection process takes place. Another cardiovascular trial provides an illustration. Timolol was one of the early beta-blocker drugs evaluated as a preventative to recurrent myocardial infarction or sudden death among heart attack survivors.[3] A large, multicenter study conducted in Norway involved 20 clinical centers that served approximately one-third of the Norwegian population. The study sample was recruited from patients admitted to these centers because of suspected acute myocardial infarction. During the enrollment period, over 11,000 subjects were considered as subjects for the trial. By the time investigators were ready to pass out pills, however, the number had been winnowed to 1884; that is, only 17% of the original sample.

Table 5–1 provides details on the reasons behind so many exclusions. By far, the largest number (about 7000) failed to meet the rather strict clinical, electrocardiographic, and serum enzyme criteria for infarction. The table includes several medical conditions as well. All this represents good experimental technique. By the time we are down to the final 1800 subjects, we have reasonable confidence that all the patients have had a heart attack. The likelihood of confounding the experiment with subjects who require multiple medications, or have other diseases, has been minimized. However, we have also eliminated many people. Some of those excluded may actually have sustained myocardial damage and others, with their multiple medical problems, may be typical of patients in many practices who might benefit from beta-blockers.

These examples highlight a major dilemma we encounter in designing and interpreting trials. The strength of the experiment is the power of the researcher to control the situation, to eliminate the extraneous, and compare

TABLE 5–1
Selection of patients for participation in the timolol study

Selection process	Number[a]
Number of screenings	11,125
Number meeting criteria for infarction	4155
Deaths before evaluation	508
Number evaluated for entry	3647
Exclusions from entry	1763 (48)
Contraindications to beta blockade	666 (18)
Serious disease impeding follow-up	260 (7)
Need for beta blockage	321 (9)
Need for other concomitant treatment	162 (4)
Administrative reasons	354 (10)
(including patient refusal)	
Randomized (participating)	1884 (52)

[a]Figures in parentheses represent percentage of 3647 patients who were evaluated for entry.
Modified, with permission, from Norwegian Multicenter Study Group.[3]

only subjects who are similar in age, sex, social status, concomitant illnesses, and medications taken. The only characteristic that should differ between the groups under study is the intervention. We want any differences in outcome that occur to be attributed to the intervention and not younger age, higher education, or fewer secondary medical conditions. The "noise" in the experiment is reduced. Factors that might confuse or dampen response are eliminated. In this ideal, experimental world, we have maximized the opportunity to get a clear, untrammeled view of the impact of the intervention. In research parlance, we are engaged in an *efficacy* trial, attempting to learn if the drug, surgical procedure, or administrative program works under ideal circumstances. Some refer to this as an *explanatory* trial. When these trials are soundly designed and executed, results are *internally valid,* meaning that within the confines of the study, results appear to be accurate and the interpretation of the investigators is supported. For the particular subjects evaluated, for example, timolol reduces future heart attacks, lovastatin is better than cholestyramine in lowering cholesterol, intrapartum fetal monitoring reduces rates of perinatal problems, or mailed patient reminders increase immunization rates. Truth is told.

However, there is a problem. In the real world things are not so tidy. Patients with heart disease may also have high blood pressure and diabetes. They may be taking an antihypertensive medication or practicing relaxation therapy. Occasionally, they do not take the pills that give them heartburn. Although the real world is not as well-controlled as experimenters would wish, this is the realm in which most of the subjects who might benefit from an intervention reside. In the timolol trial, almost 90% of the patients evaluated for entry into the trial were excluded. Many of these exclusions had to do with complexities of their medical conditions, such as other diseases and other medications. Such exclusions are good for the internal validity of the study, but sidestep reality. The question becomes, "Will results of the experiment apply to those outside this restricted sample?" Do results *generalize* to the *real world?* This notion is referred to as *external validity.* It is of considerable concern.

Even when researchers try to assemble subjects who seem typical of primary care patients, exclusion problems can become burdensome. Investigators from Seattle wished to compare physical therapy, chiropractic manipulation, and an educational booklet as treatments for patients with low back pain.[4] They conducted their study in 2 primary care clinics. Some 3800 patients were referred by their providers as potential candidates for the study. However, after these passed through the criteria gauntlet that included having pain for 7 days and no prior surgery, osteoporosis, severe concurrent illness, pregnancy, steroid therapy, prior treatment, or involvement in claims for compensation or litigation, not many were left; only 321 (8% of the potential sample) began the experiment. Again, we have a tight experimental group, but concerns as to how well the bulk of primary care patients with back pain are represented and to whom in that larger group, results of the trial may be applied.

A group from an osteoporosis center noted that recent trials of medical treatments for osteoporosis had rather strict inclusion criteria.[5] They wondered how many of the patients they routinely saw in their clinic would qualify for treatment under the research guidelines. After reviewing the charts of 420 female osteoporosis patients, they discovered that 20% or less of them would have been included. Reasons for the ineligibility appear in Table 5–2. These include being too young, too old, or too sick, or taking other medications. In 3 or 4 of the trials' criteria examined, only about 5% of the investigators' subjects would have been eligible. Explanatory power is maximized, but at a cost.

There is, not surprisingly, another side to the entry criteria coin. While strict entry criteria limit generalizability, criteria that are too loose

TABLE 5–2		
Reasons patients were not eligible for osteoporosis clinical trials		
Reason		**Percent**
Too young		28.3
Too old		7.5
Disease too severe		19.2
Comorbid condition		60.0
Cancer or cancer history	14.2	
Gastrointestinal disorders	11.7	
Rheumatic disorders	8.3	
Scoliosis	7.5	
Other conditions	25.8	
Medications		60.0
Estrogen	30.8	
Anti-osteoporosis agents	25.0	
Other medications	25.8	
All other		2.5

Modified, with permission, from Dowd, Recker, and Heaney.[5]

also extract a price. Internal validity may suffer. If many subjects who really do not have the disease under evaluation are included in a trial, results may suffer. Misclassification occurs in an unbiased or nondifferential way, but it can mask the benefits of an intervention.

Suppose, for example, that in the timolol trial, all subjects referred with a suspicion of heart attack were included. No enzyme changes or T-wave inversions were required; chest pain was enough to qualify for the study. Instead of the highly selected list of 1884 subjects, there are now over 11,000. Let's suppose that these are placed in equal portions to the timolol and placebo groups. Since most of the subjects have not had heart attacks, we should not expect them to need or to benefit from timolol. So, while a small number in each group may experience the outcome by chance (we have added 100 deaths to each group for good measure), most will not.

Table 5–3 shows that the death rate has been reduced because a large number of subjects who are much less likely to die were included. That is no surprise. More remarkable is that the difference between outcomes for the timolol and placebo groups has changed. Now, instead of a reduction of

TABLE 5–3

**Death rates (in percent) by selection criteria
for subjects receiving timolol or placebo**

Selection criteria	Number of subjects	Death rate		% reduction
		Timolol	Placebo	
Strict criteria[a]	1884	98/945 = 10.4	152/939 = 16.2	35.8
All referred subjects[b]	11,125	198/5563 = 3.6	252/5562 = 4.5	20.0

[a]Specified electrocardiographic and serum enzyme changes required.
[b]All referred patients included (hypothetical data).
Modified, with permission, from Norwegian Multicenter Study Group.[3]

almost 36% in cardiac deaths, the decline is only 20%. There is still a difference, but it has been attenuated by the inclusion of misclassified subjects. One can imagine situations where less dramatic benefits could be completely obscured by including patients who are inappropriately classified.

Subject Participation

Of the candidates who do pass muster and are eligible for a study, not everyone becomes a subject. Some folks decline to participate. One should immediately wonder, "Are nonparticipants similar to those who agree to be subjects?" Are there differences between these groups that might be important to the outcomes under study? A classic illustration of the difference between participants and nonparticipants comes from the first large-scale study that assessed the benefits of mammography.[6] In this large trial, subjects were recruited from the Health Insurance Plan (HIP) in New York City. Subjects were women between the ages of 45 and 65. Each was randomly assigned to receive either the offer of periodic mammographic screening or their "usual care." Although the study was successful in enrolling large numbers of women, not everyone who was eligible to receive mammography chose to participate. About one-third of women who were allocated to the mammography intervention were nonparticipants.

When researchers revealed the results of the study, there was a clear reduction in breast cancer mortality for women who received mammograms.

TABLE 5–4

Health Insurance Plan (HIP) of New York breast cancer screening outcomes

Deaths per 10,000 person-years		
Cause of death	Screening	Control
Breast cancer	2.6	4.1
Other cancer	16.2	17.3
Circulatory	24.0	24.9
All other causes	53.9	54.3

Modified, with permission, from Shapiro, Strax, and Venet.[6]

However, the outcomes of women who were allocated to receive mammograms but who declined the offer were also striking (Tables 5–4 and 5–5). Not only did nonparticipants have higher death rates than those who had mammograms, but the mortality experience also exceeded that of the "usual-care" comparison group. The reasons for nonparticipation were not identified, but one can imagine that prior health and associated health behaviors differed substantially and placed this group at higher risk for poor health outcomes.

Researchers responsible for executing a clinical trial on the efficacy of cholera vaccine also evaluated characteristics of nonparticipants.[7] In this

TABLE 5–5

Health Insurance Plan (HIP) of New York breast cancer screening outcomes: Participants v. nonparticipants

Deaths per 10,000 person-years			
	Screening		
Cause of death	Volunteered (2/3)	Declined (1/3)	Control
Other cancer	14.6	19.1	17.3
Circulatory	16.7	38.0	24.9
All other causes	41.5	77.4	54.3

Modified, with permission, from Shapiro, Strax, and Venet.[6]

trial, over 120,000 subjects were allocated to receive either active cholera vaccine or placebo. Again, not all those who were supposed to get the active vaccine received it. In some cases, it was because subjects refused to participate; in others, it was because they were absent at the time that the vaccine was administered in their villages. Those who refused were about 20% more likely to contract cholera than those who received placebo. For subjects who were assigned to the active vaccine group but were unavoidably absent when vaccine was administered, cholera rates were identical to those receiving placebo. In addition, investigators found that overall death rates, including those not associated with contracting cholera, were elevated among the vaccine refusers. Although when investigators compared demographic features among the placebo recipients and vaccine refusers, they could find no obvious differences, it is clear that nonparticipants carried increased risks for adverse outcomes.

ALLOCATION: SORTING SUBJECTS & CONTROLS

Subjects must be allocated by investigators. This is the activity that gives the controlled trial its special shine. However, while many people speak of the "randomized controlled trial" as if the term were all one word, random allocation of subjects is only one technique in use. As the term *random* gets tossed about rather casually, it is worth reminding ourselves precisely what it means. Randomly assigning subjects does not mean that the investigator grabs everyone sitting on the north side of the waiting room and plops them into group A, leaving folks sitting on the south side to form group B. The goal of proper subject allocation is to avoid selection bias that might create unwanted differences in comparative groups. People might congregate on the north side of the waiting room because the chairs are softer there and easier on their arthritic joints or because their friends from work sit there. Systematic differences between these people and their counterparts on the other side of the waiting room might affect results of the study. This is *convenience allocation,* and it opens the way to bias. While it may be done with best intentions of being unselective, problems can occur.

Random allocation, on the other hand, is a very carefully planned method of assigning subjects that avoids bias. It may be accomplished by making assignments from a table of random numbers, using calculator programs that generate random numbers, or even drawing numbers from a hat; but for true random assignment to take place, each subject must have an equal chance of being assigned to any of the study groups at hand. Only by using this rigorous method of allocation can we guard against the unconscious biases of the assigning investigators and, indeed, the study subjects themselves.

Nonrandom Allocation

An example of biased allocation comes from a study that attempted to assess the risks and benefits of delivering babies in a special birthing room.[8] In this experiment, 500 women were offered the chance to deliver in a "bedroom-type room next to the delivery suite." Amenities included a queen-sized bed, casual furnishings, and a large private bathroom. Also included in the birthing-room delivery plan was a series of agreements between patients and staff that included avoidance of intravenous fluids, fetal monitors, excessive analgesia, and much of the paraphernalia associated with traditional in-hospital deliveries. The patients participating in this birthing-room experience were compared with a "similar number of low-risk mothers and babies in the standard delivery room." The results of the study suggest not only that the birthing room was safe but also that deliveries occurring there had fewer complications for mother and baby than deliveries under standard conditions. The author evaluated 42 perinatal outcomes in the 2 groups and found that birthing-room deliveries had a significantly lower rate for 12 complications, including those listed in Table 5–6.

The author registers happy surprise at what he terms the "unexpected" results; but the reduced rate of complications in the experimental group is probably not unexpected. Let us review exactly how subjects were allocated to the birthing-room and standard-care groups. Participants in the birthing-room deliveries were volunteers. Women in the standard-care group declined the birthing-room offer for reasons that are not clearly specified.

Are the groups comparable? Are the risks that may influence the outcome of pregnancy equivalent in both? We know that the patients differ in one important respect: one group volunteered to participate in the birthing-room experiment, while the other did not wish to partake. Could this difference affect results? We are supplied with little information about

TABLE 5-6

Complication rates for standard delivery v. alternative birthing center (ABC)

	Standard delivery (% of cases)	ABC (% of cases)
Labor		
Failure to progress	18.3	5.2
C-section	9.2	2.3
Fetal distress	5.3	0.3
Meconium staining	11.9	2.3
Infant		
Child abuse	2.4	0
Congenital anomalies	3.0	0.6
Jaundice	12.6	2.4

Modified, with permission, from Goodlin.[8]

characteristics of these two groups of women that might help us decide. However, we know enough about volunteers in health programs to make a guess that the birthing-room volunteers were probably somewhat older, better educated, and of higher socioeconomic status and parity than the comparison women. Since these factors are known to be associated with a favorable outcome of pregnancy, we have a situation where the intervention, the birthing room, appears to produce lower complication rates when, in fact, improved outcomes are a manifestation of allocating a healthier group of women to the experimental group. The fact that infant outcomes such as child abuse and anomalies are *not* likely to be related to the birthing room, supports an alternative explanation. Women interested in birthing rooms will probably produce bigger, bouncier babies regardless of the type of delivery employed.

Had the author of this study randomly allocated only subjects who were willing to undergo the birthing-room experience, patient-selection biases might have been avoided and the results might have been very different. An elegance of allocation is illustrated in a Canadian study on a similar subject.[9] Investigators in this report wished to explore the possible benefits of the Leboyer approach to childbirth, a method that promotes birth in a dark, quiet room, delayed clamping of the umbilical cord, and calming of the infant by massage and bathing in warm water. To guard against lack of comparability between the Leboyer and "conventional delivery" groups, all subjects were required to fulfill eligibility requirements that included a low obstetrical risk score and interest in the Leboyer approach to childbirth before they were entered in the study. Random assignment was then made, so that each woman had an equal chance of having her infant delivered by the Leboyer or conventional method. As things turned out, the authors were unable to demonstrate any important advantage to soft lights and tepid baths when compared with a conventional albeit gentle delivery.

Historic Controls

A common method of *control* is to compare results from experimental subjects with outcomes from patients treated before the new intervention was available. These are *historic controls*, and the design is sometimes referred to as a *before-and-after* study. The technique has considerable "curbside appeal." Investigators note the rates of a disease prior to the initiation of an intervention, then reassess and note beneficial changes in the aftermath. Sometimes this involves different subject groups measured at two points in time, or the same subjects can be measured twice, thus serving as their own controls. The approach can be quite efficient and, if the same subjects are followed before and after treatment, the comparability of control subjects is assured.

Some years ago, when researchers from Minnesota wanted to test a vaccine against the common cold, subjects became their own controls.[10] Students from the university were asked to volunteer for the study if they were known to be "particularly susceptible to colds." Subjects supplied baseline information regarding the frequency and symptoms of colds in the preceding year; they were then given vaccine, and instructed to report to the health service whenever a cold developed. The reduction in colds experienced following immunization was remarkable. Subjects had reported an average of 5.9 colds in the year preceding vaccination. During the study year, only 1.6 per subject were documented. Sounds like victory over a major human nemesis.

But these investigators punctured their own balloon. Not content to rely on the before-and-after comparison, they included a concurrent, randomly assigned group of subjects from the same student pool who were given saline injections instead of vaccine. This other, randomly assigned, control group reported an average of 5.6 colds in the year preceding inoculation and 2.1 colds per subject in their "post-vaccination" year—practically speaking, the same results as the active vaccination group.

Why should such a decline in colds occur? Several factors may be at play, and each points to a frailty of the historic control approach. To begin with, things change over time. In particular, infectious diseases vary from season to season. It is possible that in the year preceding the vaccination experiment, Minnesota had a particularly bad season for colds. In the follow-up year, there were fewer viruses in the community. One can also imagine reporting bias creeping in. Recall that the number of colds experienced by each subject in the year preceding immunization was self-reported, whereas colds in the year following immunization were documented by the health service. There is certainly room for exaggerating the past, especially if selective recall might get you into a study that was likely to benefit your health.

There is also the likely occurrence of a phenomenon known as *regression to the mean*. Regression occurs when subjects are selected for study on the basis of extreme values of a risk factor, such as very high blood pressure or cholesterol level or low white blood cell count. Remeasurements of subjects' values are likely to be less extreme, that is, they regress or move toward the average of the population, regardless of any treatment or change in their condition.

Before-and-after study problems are not limited to studies of infectious diseases. Difficulties with the technique were discovered in the early chapters of the unhappy story of diethylstilbestrol (DES). This hormone was believed at one time to prevent recurrent abortion in pregnant women. It was administered to women who had lost previous pregnancies in the expectation that the steroid would help them carry to term. The practice proliferated after reports of dramatically improved outcomes for DES-treated pregnancies compared with outcomes for prior pregnancies.[11] Table 5–7 shows these results.

TABLE 5–7

Pregnancy outcomes of women with habitual abortion after treatment with diethylstilbestrol (DES)

	Patients	Pregnancies	Living infants	Success rate, %
Prior pregnancies	38	174	15	8.5
Study pregnancy	38	42	19	45.2

Modified, with permission, from Davis and Fugo.[11]

Promising as the findings appear, the value of DES did not hold up. Dieckmann et al criticized the earlier work for "lack of adequate control."[12] They suggested that patients receiving the trial medication also received more meticulous medical care and attention than they had with previous pregnancies. Factors other than DES may have been responsible for the improved outcomes. When these authors compared outcomes of pregnant women given DES with those of women treated *simultaneously* whose management was similar in every way except that a placebo pill was given in place of the active hormone, the benefits of DES vanished. The unfortunate long-term sequel to this story was not only that DES did not improve pregnancy outcomes, but, some years later, caused an epidemic of cancer in female offspring of women who received the treatment.

Randomized Controls

Random allocation is the method of choice for controlled trials. However, even when this is executed properly, there is a risk that randomization will not accomplish its intended purpose. Random assignment attempts to equalize experimental and comparison groups by giving each subject an equal chance to be in any of the groups. But chance is chancy business, as anyone who has flipped coins or played cards can avow. Just as it is possible to come up with heads for 8 out of 10 flips of the coin, so can groups assigned by the random process turn out to be dissimilar in their makeup.

Investigators should check to see whether random assignments result in comparable groups. A table displaying baseline characteristics of subjects according to their treatment group is an essential part of the report of a randomized trial. Table 5–8 gives an example from the timolol trial.[3] Along with standard demographic variables such as age and sex, tables such as this one should include variables that might influence the outcome. In the timolol example, risk factors, such as smoking, measures of cardiac function, and location of infarct, all are important to consider. Review of the table suggests that the random allocation process worked. The timolol and placebo groups appear to be balanced.

Such success is not always achieved, however. When researchers in Edinburgh attempted to assess the efficacy of a practice-based breast cancer detection program, their units of random allocation were 87 general practices in the Edinburgh vicinity.[13] Intervention practices were to provide annual breast examinations and biannual mammography to female patients between the ages of 45 and 64. Control practices provided women with

TABLE 5–8

Characteristics of 1884 randomized patients in the timolol trial before treatment

	Treatment group	
	Placebo (n = 939)	Timolol (n = 945)
	%	
Sex		
Men	78	80
Women	22	20
Age		
<64 years	59	63
65–75 years	41	37
Clinical history		
Previous infarction	19	19
Angina	38	38
Treated hypertension	22	18
Smoking	53	54
Therapy before admission		
Digitalis	14	15
Diuretics	23	18
Beta-blockers	10	10
Risk factors for this study		
Heart failure	34	32
Enlarged heart	23	21
Lowest systolic blood pressure (<100 mmHg)	25	23
Atrial fibrillation or flutter	12	11

Modified, with permission from Norwegian Multicenter Study Group.[3]

their "usual care." The reasons practices rather than individuals were randomized were several: many of the physicians in the study were unwilling to offer breast cancer detection services to some but not all patients in the practice. It was also recognized that patients talk to one another and that differential treatment would certainly arouse concerns. So, *cluster allocation* in such a situation makes sense; the practices rather than patients become the units randomly assigned to experimental and control conditions.

Investigators trust that any characteristics of patients within the practices that might be related to outcome will be equally distributed.

Unfortunately, such was not the case. Some characteristics of the practices were comparable—the age distributions, for example. But one important factor, socioeconomic status (SES), was badly unbalanced. Practices serving women of higher SES had much greater representation in the experimental, screening group. Researchers worried that this imbalance could influence the results. SES is known as a predictor of health outcomes and could influence mortality in the 2 groups and confuse the assessment of the impact of the intervention. Solving this comparability problem was challenging. Eventually the investigators devised detailed classification systems for SES and used statistical models to perform post hoc adjustments on the data. Evidence that the unbalanced allocation was influencing results was confirmed. After adjustment for SES, a 21% reduction in deaths attributed to the screening program was observed compared to the unadjusted estimate of only 13%.[14]

Bias can occur any time groups being compared are unequal with respect to either risk factors that predispose to disease or existing conditions that may influence outcome. While there are methods for dealing with unanticipated inequalities when data are analyzed, most investigators would rather not be victimized by the noncomparability problem in the first place. If important risk factors or *comorbid conditions* (concurrent illnesses that may influence outcome) can be identified at the outset, subjects may be grouped or prognostically stratified prior to assignment.

In the Leboyer childbirth example, the investigators were savvy enough to use prognostic stratification to avoid the pitfalls of this multi-risk situation. Before assignment, patients were grouped according to parity and social class, and random allocation proceeded separately within each subgroup. The likelihood that high-risk first pregnancies will end up being compared with less risky subsequent pregnancies because of chance maldistribution is thus minimized.

Blinding

The tidiest of unbiased allocations can come undone if subjects or investigators have knowledge of the assignments. An endearing frailty of our species is our strong desire for things to turn out well. This desire is as strong in medical research as in any endeavor. Both investigators and subjects want treatments to work. This means that an essential ingredient of any randomized trial is a plan to keep both those who receive and those who administer and measure the outcomes of an intervention as protected from potential bias as possible. *Double blinding* in a study means that assignments have been concealed from both subjects and investigators.

Schulz et al supported the importance of this when they reviewed 250 controlled trials from the pregnancy and childbirth literature.[15] They found that trials in which concealment of treatment allocation was inadequate or poorly described had exaggerated estimates of treatment effects compared with trials that reported adequate concealment. Such blinding is, of course, much easier with pills than it is with surgical procedures, birthing rooms, or administrative interventions.

Evidence that investigators have gone to whatever lengths to promote treatment concealment is a positive. In a multicenter trial evaluating an oral chelating agent known as succimer for treating elevated lead levels in children, investigators worried that the strong, unpleasant sulfur aroma of the drug would not only foil concealment but reduce its palatability among the young subjects.[16] Accordingly, they impregnated the bottle cap of the placebo capsules with a similarly noxious sulfur smell in the hopes of maintaining "blindness." This noble effort was only partially successful. The phony aroma in the bottle cap fooled some but not all of the toddlers. When adherence rates to the medication were recorded, fewer doses of the succimer were administered than placebo.

FOLLOW-UP

The best-laid plans—selecting, allocating, and assessing subjects—come to little if the experiment fails in its execution. Subjects need to take their pills, adhere to their diets, or follow the practice guidelines being evaluated. Researchers need to keep track of subjects so that proper assessment of outcomes can occur. Attention to issues of adherence and attrition is vital to study validity of both the internal and external sorts.

Adherence

It seems self-evident that if subjects do not follow the intervention to which they have been assigned, we are in for trouble. One cannot tell whether lovastatin reduces cholesterol if folks will not take it, or whether nicotine patches curtail cigarette smoking if subjects do not wear them. If overall rates of compliance are low for all methods under scrutiny, beneficial effects of any of the agents may be masked. Treatment of high blood pressure has always been plagued by compliance problems; people with asymptomatic conditions have a difficult time remembering to take their pills. Suppose we were trying to compare a new antihypertensive agent with one of the standard treatments available. Both medications are tablets that are taken twice daily. Neither medication has an offensive taste or intolerable side effects. In other words, we anticipate no difference in compliance. However, it turns out that the patients we are studying are very relaxed about taking their prescribed medications. When it comes to looking at the results, we find little improvement in the control of high blood pressure among patients taking the new agent compared with those taking the old therapy. However, we also discover that only 20% of patients took their pills regularly. Under these circumstances, it is very difficult to know whether or not the drug under study has a beneficial effect. As in the timolol example, where medication effects could be diluted by including improperly diagnosed heart attack patients, low overall compliance may hide a real benefit.

One approach to reducing the problems created by nonadherence is to nip it in the bud. Investigators in the Physicians' Health Study built a "run-in phase" into their design.[2] The 33,000 physicians who were deemed eligible for the study were given aspirin for several months before randomization took place. The idea was to muster out those who could not tolerate aspirin because of adverse effects or who took their medicine less than two-thirds of the time. By the time the run-in phase had been completed, only 22,000 doctor subjects were left. The run-in served its purpose, however. After 5 years of follow-up, 99% of the physicians were still providing information to researchers, and over 80% continued to take their pills. The study identified a 44% reduction in heart attack risk among this highly selected group. Under these ideal circumstances, aspirin works. Unfortunately, in the real world, issues of noncompliance and adverse effects do exist, casting some doubt on the overall *effectiveness* of the aspirin intervention.

Factoring adherence into assessments is not as simple as it might appear. Investigators from the Coronary Drug Project Research Group found little difference in the 5-year mortality from heart disease among men given the lipid-lowering drug clofibrate compared with those given placebo.[17] Death rates were about 20% in both groups over the 5-year study. Recognizing that not all subjects were likely to adhere to a regimen that required gulping 3 capsules 3 times a day, researchers counted remaining capsules each time subjects returned for a follow-up visit. They were then able to distinguish subjects who were "good adherers" and took more than 80% of their allotted pills from those who were not so faithful. When they checked mortality against adherence, the results were dramatic. As seen in Table 5–9, the mortality for those who took their pills was only 15% compared with almost 25% for nonadherers. It appears that differential adherence is masking a substantial treatment benefit. But adherence data were also available on placebo takers. And, as the right-hand column of Table 5–9 indicates, differential mortality among adherers and nonadherers to placebo was almost identical to that of those who took clofibrate.

This is sobering news indeed. It suggests that health risks related to important outcomes, such as mortality, differ between those who take and those who do not take medications regardless of the biologic activity of the drug.

Differential compliance can occur if treatments being compared place unequal demands on subjects. When Deyo and colleagues wanted to test the optimal duration of bed rest as a treatment for low back pain, they

TABLE 5–9

Five-year mortality in patients given clofibrate or placebo, according to cumulative adherence to protocol prescription

	Treatment group			
	Clofibrate		Placebo	
Adherence[a]	No. of patients	% mortality[b]	No. of patients	% mortality[b]
<80%	357	24.6 ± 2.3 (22.5)	882	28.2 ± 1.5 (25.8)
≥80%	708	15.0 ± 1.3 (15.7)	1813	15.1 ± 0.8 (16.4)
Total study group	1065	18.2 ± 1.2 (18.0)	2695	19.4 ± 0.8 (19.5)

[a]A patient's cumulative adherence was computed as the estimated number of capsules actually taken as a percentage of the number that should have been taken according to the protocol during the first 5 years of follow-up or until death (if death occurred during the first 5 years).
[b]The figures in parentheses are adjusted for 40 baseline characteristics. The figures given as percentages ± 1 standard error (SE) are unadjusted figures, the SEs of which are correct to within 0.1 unit for the adjusted figures.
Modified, with permission, from Coronary Drug Project Research Group.[17]

anticipated adherence differences in their 2-day versus 7-day bed rest regimens.[18] As they suspected, not all subjects followed instructions. Some lingered in bed for more time than they were allotted, and some for less. Lapses were greater in the 7-day subjects. The group assigned to 2 days of rest averaged 2.3 days in bed while the 7-day group averaged less than 4. About three-quarters of 7-day subjects reported that they actually spent less than 7 days in bed. When the researchers found little difference in symptoms, signs, or functional status at the 3-week follow-up visit, they worried that differential compliance might have masked a difference in outcomes. So they restricted their analysis to subjects who followed bed rest instructions most closely. There was still no difference in perceptions of pain or general well-being. The one clear difference between the 2 bed rest regimens that did appear was that those in the 2-day group missed much less work than those assigned to rest for 7 days, about 2 days less on average. The authors concluded that "less is more." Productivity can be preserved with less extensive care.

Sometimes problems of adherence become more evident with time. In such instances, planning an evaluation that is of sufficient duration is essential to assessing value. When investigators sought data on potential benefits of a low-carbohydrate (Atkins type) diet on achieving weight loss, they randomly assigned 132 markedly obese individuals to either a low-fat or low-carbohydrate diet.[19] Researchers found that over the 6-month study interval the low-carbohydrate dieters shed significantly more pounds than their low-fat diet compatriots. There were hints, however, that the good news should be viewed with some reserve. Only 79 of the 132 (60%) subjects who began the trial were still on their diets by 6 months, suggesting that long-term success of both diets might be in question.

Indeed, a companion article in the same journal issue reported on a similar diet comparison of 1 year duration.[20] This experiment also compared weight loss among low-carbohydrate and low-fat dieters (33 and 30 subjects, respectively, in each group). By 6 months into the study, 42 of the 63 subjects (67%) remained on their diets and findings favored the low-carbohydrate group. They had an average weight loss of 7%, more than twice as much as the comparison group. By 12 months, however, results were less robust. Only 37 subjects were still on their diets. The low-carbohydrate, Atkins-type dieters had slipped to an average weight loss of only 4.4% from baseline values compared with an average loss of 2.5% for the low-fat group. The difference between the two was no longer deemed significant (more about this in Chapter 8). Because obesity, like other chronic health conditions, requires remedies that can be sustained over the long term (indeed over a lifetime), evaluations of short-run efficacy where there is little prospect of long-term adherence may offer little.

Attrition

Anytime subjects are lost to follow-up, whether in observational or experimental studies, valuable information may be lost. The worry is that attrition occurs differentially and will bias outcomes. During the timolol trial, a number of patients withdrew during the course of the study. Although some of these defections were for nonmedical reasons, many were due to adverse reactions that could be drug related. Over the course of the trial, 26% of the 1884 subjects withdrew. These withdrawals were not evenly divided among placebo and timolol recipients. More timolol subjects left the study and a greater proportion of these withdrew in the first month of follow-up. Table 5–10 indicates some of the reasons for withdrawal. Greater numbers of individuals taking timolol experienced hypotension and low heart rate than those taking placebo, and they left the study. These factors could influence results. Patients experiencing such adverse reactions might also be more susceptible to cardiac outcomes. If more

TABLE 5–10
Withdrawal from treatment for adverse reactions among 1884 patients given timolol or placebo

	No. of patients	
Category of reaction	Placebo 939	Timolol 945
Cardiac failure, nonfatal	20	27
Pulmonary edema, nonfatal	2	8
Heart rate < 40 beats/min	2	37
Hypotension	11	26
Claudication	3	13
Bronchial obstruction	4	10
Cerebrovascular disease	6	10

Modified, with permission, from Norwegian Multicenter Study Group.[3]

timolol subjects who are likely to have an adverse event drop out, the drug will appear in a more favorable light than is warranted.

This situation presents a dilemma to investigators. If results for only those who stay in the study are analyzed, biased withdrawal can create the unwarranted impression of benefit. On the other hand, continuing to count subjects as in the trial when they drop out after a month or two and no longer receive benefits of the medication seems inappropriate. What is one to do? The Norwegian investigators took an approach that has become the norm. It is known as analysis by *intention to treat.* This means that subjects are analyzed according to the categories into which they were originally randomized. If subjects withdraw because of adverse effects, or fail to take their pills, or stay on bed rest for longer or shorter periods of time than they were assigned, it does not matter. They belong to their original treatment allocation.

When the timolol study investigators looked at the outcomes of all their subjects by intention to treat, they found that 142 of the 900 subjects in the placebo group had suffered cardiac death compared with only 83 of 900 who received timolol (see Table 5–11). They also restricted the analysis to deaths that occurred during or soon after patients stopped treatment. Results were similar. The benefits of timolol held up when only subjects on treatment were considered, as well as by intention to treat.

	Deaths	
	Placebo ($n = 939$)	Timolol ($n = 945$)
During or within 28 days of end of treatment		
Sudden cardiac	95	47
All cardiac	113	58
All deaths	117	67
During treatment	98	15
Within 28 days of end of treatment	19	12
After 28 days withdrawal from treatment		
Total	**152**	**98**

TABLE 5–11
Outcomes of timolol trial by treatment status

Modified, with permission, from Norwegian Multicenter Study Group.[3]

When results withstand this double scrutiny, confidence in the validity of findings is enhanced. The benefits of a treatment are more difficult to demonstrate with intention-to-treat analyses. Including subjects who are unlikely to have experienced benefit from the intervention mitigates differences.

ANALYSIS

Competing Interventions

In some intervention studies, particularly those in which a subject's behavior is the target of treatment, the risk to validity is not that intervention subjects do not comply with treatment but that control subjects do. If members of the comparison group change their habits in a manner that lowers risk for the outcome of concern, apparent benefits of intervention may be diminished or even lost. A well-known example comes from the large multiple-risk factor intervention trial known as MRFIT.[21] This ambitious project evaluated the effects of reducing high blood pressure, elevated cholesterol, and cigarette smoking on rates of cardiovascular disease. Over 12,000 men who were determined to be at high risk from some combination of these risk factors were assigned to either a "special-intervention" or a "usual-care" group. Special-intervention subjects had diet counseling to lower their cholesterol, were placed in smoking cessation programs, and underwent medical protocols to reduce their elevated blood pressures. Usual-care subjects were referred back to their regular health providers.

Subjects in both groups were followed up for an average of 7 years. At completion of the trial, rates of death from coronary heart disease, cardiovascular disease, and all causes were compared. Heart disease and cardiovascular deaths were reduced among special-intervention subjects by 7.1 and 4.7%, respectively, a slight and not statistically significant improvement. The overall death rate of the special-intervention group was actually a few percentage points higher—rather disappointing results after 10 years of effort!

Investigators offered several interpretations of these findings. The first, of course, was the possibility that the intervention simply had no effect on mortality. However, a second possibility was that the benefits may have been masked by an unanticipated improvement in the risk profiles of the usual-care subjects. During the time the trial was in progress, there was widespread media coverage that created increasing awareness about the risks of smoking and high cholesterol levels. Many individuals began to curtail their cigarette smoking, improve their exercise habits, and reduce dietary fat on their own. The "usual-care" group was susceptible to this information blitz, a *cointervention* over which investigators had no control.

Indeed, the control subjects had, as a group, lowered their blood pressures, reduced their smoking, and dropped their cholesterol levels over the course of the trial. While their improvements were not as great as those in the special-intervention group, the risk reduction appeared sufficient to obscure the benefits of the interventions. The fact that death rates for both groups were substantially lower than had been predicted at the start of the trial lends support to this theory. On the basis of best estimates available, when the trial began, investigators anticipated a coronary heart disease death rate of 29 per 1000. In fact, mortality from coronary heart disease was 18 per 1000 in the special-intervention group and 19 per 1000 among the usual-care subjects.

Outcomes/End Points

Readers should give some thought to the "end points" or outcomes that are reported in clinical trials. Are the effects of the intervention clearly defined? Are they comparably determined? Do the end points selected include the most important possible outcomes of the trial? Several trials that have shown promise in reducing mortality from a specific cause have been disappointing when deaths from other causes were considered.

The remarkable advance in treatment of coronary artery disease brought about by the use of coronary stents has been hampered by the problem of restenosis. The prospect that renarrowing of the artery due to cellular buildup within these implanted wire tubes might be avoided by radiation was investigated in a randomized trial.[22] Researchers allocated 252 subjects to receive either an indwelling intracoronary ribbon that contained small radioactive seeds or a similar-appearing nonradioactive device. The designated primary end points for the study were "a composite of death, myocardial infarction, and the need for repeated re-vascularization of the target lesion."[22] After 9 months of follow-up, findings appeared promising. Forty-four percent of subjects given the placebo ribbon had experienced target end points compared with only 28% of those in the radioactive group. However, closer scrutiny reveals that not all end points are created equal. The major benefits of the therapy were, as anticipated, a reduced need to perform additional revascularizing procedures on subjects who had received radiation. The other end points, death and myocardial infarction, were not so favorably distributed. Three percent of patients who received radiation died and 10% had heart attacks compared with only 1 and 4%, respectively, in the placebo group. The radiation appeared to achieve its early objective of reducing new cellular growth at the site of the stent. However, the later complications of the procedure are more important outcomes, and their increased occurrence among the patients receiving radiation suggests that more work is needed.

In the timolol study, researchers recognized the possibility that the beta-blocker could have a beneficial effect on the outcomes of recurrent heart attack and sudden cardiac death but cause problems in other domains. So they assessed both the target outcomes and overall mortality. Figure 5–2 shows a *life-table* analysis, also known as *survival analysis,* for both cardiac event deaths and all-cause mortality. Survival analysis is a particularly useful way of comparing the occurrence of medical events over time. The technique acknowledges that the number of subjects in a trial changes as deaths occur, new subjects are recruited into the study, or folks leave town or decide they no longer wish to participate. Survival analysis continually adjusts for these perturbations and gives credit to subjects for the time they are active participants in the trial. As the figures indicate, timolol held up, reducing deaths from cardiac events and all causes.

Consider which end points are meaningful. When a Utah law was passed requiring training of individuals who serve alcohol in restaurants and bars to provide "more responsible beverage service," an experiment was conducted to assess the effects of the intervention.[23] In all, 97 servers and 43 managers, representing 26 establishments, took part in a 1-day training session. For comparison, 14 establishments of similar size and type where training had not yet occurred were selected. Participants completed pre- and postsession questionnaires that measured their beliefs and knowledge about responsible alcohol service. One month following the education program, trained observers visited the establishments to observe actual practice.

The pencil-and-paper results were encouraging. Servers and managers demonstrated better knowledge and attitudes about responsible serving practices. Unfortunately, behavior did not follow suit. No differences were noted between intervention and control establishments in the ways in which servers communicated with customers or limited the delivery of drinks.

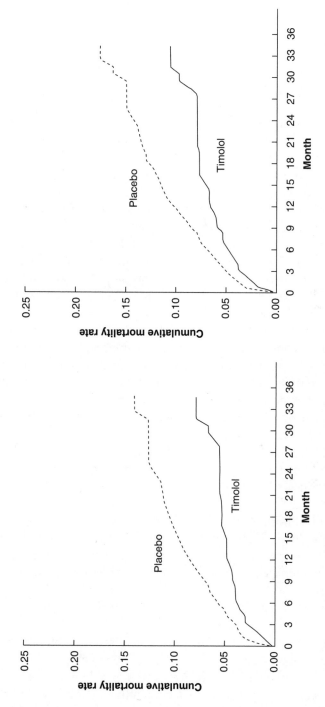

FIGURE 5–2. Left: Life-table cumulated rates of sudden cardiac death during administration of medication or within 28 days of the last dose. **Right:** Life-table cumulated rates of death from all causes. These deaths occurred while patients were taking the test medication or within 28 days of administration of last dose. (Modified, with permission, from Norwegian Multicenter Study Group.[3])

SCOPE

Although the randomized clinical trial (RCT) design is generally employed to determine whether treatments are beneficial, sometimes other useful information can emerge. A trial intended to evaluate the efficacy of an intervention can turn up findings on adverse consequences as a bonus. An experiment created to test the benefits of the inhibitor of the enzyme, cyclooxygenase-2 or COX-2, on the recurrence of colorectal polyps is an example.[24] Celecoxib, one of the class of COX-2 inhibitors, appeared to have the potential to prevent the formation of adenomas of the colon and rectum. Accordingly, a trial was initiated in which over 2000 patients with a history of polyps were randomly assigned to 1 of 3 groups: placebo, celecoxib 200 mg twice daily or celecoxib 400 mg twice daily. Because there had been reports of excess adverse events such as heart attack and stroke associated with COX-2 inhibitors, cardiovascular safety was also monitored.

Not all the subjects had completed the 3-year study when disturbing findings emerged. Those in the 200-mg celecoxib group were more than twice as likely to die from a cardiovascular cause or experience a nonfatal myocardial infarction, stroke, or heart failure as those taking placebo; those in the higher dose celecoxib group had three times the risk. In response, the investigators elected to discontinue the study medications among subjects who had not completed the trial.

The clinical trial has also been used to assess directly the problem of adverse effects. When a nonabsorbable fat was developed as a substitute for the triglycerides that make snack foods like potato chips so irresistible, it seemed a dieter's dream come true—fewer calories consumed with less fat too. Unfortunately, olestra had not been on the market long before reports of unpleasant effects began to appear. Numerous complaints of bloating, gas, and diarrhea were registered. But were these occurring at a rate that was greater than one would expect in the normal course of events?

To answer the question investigators went to a suburban Chicago multiplex cinema to conduct an ingenious trial.[25] Over 1000 adult and teenage moviegoers were offered free passes to a first-run motion picture. They were then randomized to receive a bag of potato chips made either with olestra or with standard triglyceride as well as a 32 ounce beverage. They were allowed to consume as much or as little of the chips and drink as they desired. About 2 days after the theater experience participants were

TABLE 5–12			
Adverse gastrointestinal (GI) events reported after eating potato chips made with triglyceride or olestra (in percent)			

	Treatment group	
	Triglyceride	Olestra
Adverse event	($n = 529$)	($n = 563$)
Any GI event	17.6	15.8
Gas	6.4	4.8
Diarrhea	2.6	3.0
Abdominal pain	3.6	2.3
Upset stomach	2.1	2.0
Abdominal cramping	1.9	2.0
Loose stools	1.1	1.6
Other GI events[a]	4.0	3.4

[a]Other GI events include nausea, bloating, indigestion, aftertaste, belching, constipation, vomiting, or bloody stool.
Modified, with permission, from Cheskin et al.[25]

queried by telephone about any digestive symptoms they had encountered in the interval. The results are illustrated in Table 5–12. A remarkable number of subjects reported gastrointestinal disturbances—more than 15% in each group. However, no difference in symptoms was observed between those eating the olestra and those consuming the triglyceride chips.

SUMMARY

This all seems a tremendous effort to expend just looking at the methods of controlled trials, but by now certain principles should have a familiar ring. The problems of comparability of comparison subjects and the forces of selection that go into choosing exposed or experimental subjects have come up before in discussing case-control and follow-up designs. The principles are the same. The reader has a right to expect an author to supply the information necessary to generalize from the specific study to other populations. We can likewise expect that care has been used in selecting comparison subjects, and that when questions of comparability arise, the author will provide information about how subjects and their controls are similar and how they differ.

Although experimental designs, like follow-up studies, are not encumbered by recall bias and problems encountered in using data from the past, they share the plague of attrition. Both of these prospective designs depend on following up on subjects over time to assess outcomes. The risk that patients will drop out of the project because they experience adverse effects from a medication or are unable to comply with a complicated diet is a constant threat to results.

Comfort in assessing these methodological pitfalls comes only with practice—reading many studies and scouring the methodology for problems. But remember, flaw catching can become a disheartening addiction, since very few studies are free of blemish. If you look hard enough, weakness may be found in the most robust of designs. We must guard against dismissing a study because of defects that are relatively unimportant. When flaws are found, we must ask whether the problems will impinge on the validity of the study. In cases such as the birthing-room experiment, where great potential for bias exists from the unequal distribution of risk factors in the two groups, the problem is crippling. After assessing this design, one would do well to proceed to other reading tasks. In other cases, such as the differential compliance seen in the study on bed rest for low back pain, the potential threat probably did not have a major impact on results.

Investigators, like the rest of us, are subject to the imperfections of humanity. They concoct and serve up their studies with the best of intentions. Often the seasoning is not quite right, and sometimes critical ingredients are missing or misapportioned. Have compassion for the cooks; try to distinguish between small matters of taste and major indigestibilities.

REFERENCES

1. Moher D, Schulz KF, Altman D: The CONSORT statement: Revised recommendations for improving the quality of reports of parallel-group randomized trials. JAMA 2001;285(15):1987.
2. Steering Committee of the Physicians' Health Study Research Group: Final report on the aspirin component of the ongoing Physicians' Health Study. N Engl J Med 1989;321(3):129.

3. Norwegian Multicenter Study Group: Timolol-induced reduction in mortality and reinfarction in patients surviving acute myocardial infarction. N Engl J Med 1981;304(14):801.

4. Cherkin DC et al: A comparison of physical therapy, chiropractic manipulation, and provision of an educational booklet for the treatment of patients with low back pain. N Engl J Med 1998;339(15):1021.

5. Dowd R, Recker RR, Heaney RP: Study subjects and ordinary patients. Osteoporosis Int 2000;11(6):533.

6. Shapiro S, Strax P, Venet L: Periodic breast cancer screening in reducing mortality from breast cancer. JAMA 1971;215(11):1777.

7. Clemens JD et al: Nonparticipation as a determinant of adverse health outcomes in a field trial of oral cholera vaccines. Am J Epidemiol 1992; 135(8):865.

8. Goodlin RC: Low-risk obstetric care for low-risk mothers. Lancet 1980; 1:1017.

9. Nelson NM et al: A randomized clinical trial of the Leboyer approach to childbirth. N Engl J Med 1980;302:655.

10. Diehl HS, Baker AB, Cowan DW: Cold vaccines: An evaluation based on a controlled study. JAMA 1938;111:1168.

11. Davis ME, Fugo NW: Early pregnancy complications. JAMA 1950;142: 778.

12. Dieckmann WJ et al: Does the administration of diethylstilbestrol during pregnancy have therapeutic value? Am J Obstet Gynecol 1953;66:1062.

13. Alexander F et al: Randomisation by cluster and the problem of social class bias. J Epidemiol Community Health 1989;43(1):29.

14. Alexander FE et al: 14 years of follow-up from the Edinburgh randomised trial of breast-cancer screening. Lancet 1999;353(9168):1903.

15. Schulz KF et al: Empirical evidence of bias: Dimensions of methodological quality associated with estimates of treatment effects in controlled trials. JAMA 1995;273(5):408.

16. Rogan WJ et al: The effect of chelation therapy with succimer on neuropsychological development in children exposed to lead. N Engl J Med 2001;344(19):1421.

17. Coronary Drug Project Research Group: Influence of adherence to treatment and response of cholesterol on mortality in the coronary drug project. N Engl J Med 1980;303(18):1038.

18. Deyo R, Diehl A, Rosenthal M: How many days of bed rest for acute low back pain. N Engl J Med 1986;315(17):1064.

19. Samaha FF et al. A low-carbohydrate as compared with a low-fat diet in severe obesity. N Engl J Med 2003;348:2074.

20. Foster GD et al. A randomized trial of a low-carbohydrate diet for obesity. N Engl J Med 2003;348:2082.

21. Multiple Risk Factor Intervention Trial Research Group: Multiple risk factor intervention trial: Risk factor changes and mortality results. JAMA 1982;248:1465.

22. Leon MB et al: Localized intracoronary gamma-radiation therapy to inhibit the recurrence of restenosis after stenting. N Engl J Med 2001;344(4):250.

23. Howard-Pitney B et al: Responsible alcohol service: A study of server, manager, and environmental impact. Am J Public Health 1991;81:197.

24. Solomon SD et al: Cardiovascular risk associated with celecoxib in a clinical trial for colorectal adenoma prevention. N Engl J Med 2005;352:1071.

25. Cheskin LJ et al: Gastrointestinal symptoms following consumption of olestra or regular triglyceride potato chips; a controlled comparison. JAMA 1998;279:150.

CHAPTER SIX

Study Design: Variations

A foolish consistency is the hobgoblin of little minds.

R. W. EMERSON

We have laid out a menu of study designs. Each entrée has distinctive ingredients that give it texture, flavor, and its own value in a balanced diet. Each design has different occasions on which it is best served. However, some flexibility is required: Our first choice is not always available. Several limitations can constrain investigators. Even when we are fully aware of the strongest methodological approach to a problem, other considerations may prompt other choices. This is particularly true when we come to evaluating interventions, an activity that is taking up larger and larger slices of journal space.

In this chapter, we will retreat somewhat from the impression left in Chapter 5, that the only acceptable way to evaluate an intervention—be it pill, procedure, pamphlet, or policy—is through the randomized controlled trial (RCT). The RCT is certainly the strongest design we have examined up to now, but for a variety of reasons, it is not always the dish of choice. Some of these reasons include *real-world considerations, practical constraints*, and *ethical concerns*. This chapter will give us an opportunity to review some features of designs we have covered so far. In addition, we will explore some new uses for old friends. New applications may appear incongruent with the admonitions of earlier chapters, but as Emerson suggests, the expansive mind can cope with a bit of inconsistency.

REAL-WORLD CONSIDERATIONS

Much was made in the preceding chapter of the trade-off between tight control of trials to maximize explanatory power and the ability to generalize study findings to broader populations. We called it internal versus external validity. Adhering to strict diagnostic criteria, minimizing "noise," or confusing variables that might be introduced by subjects who had multiple medical conditions or who were involved in other interventions, and improving compliance through run-in periods were techniques that gave an intervention the optimal chance to "strut its stuff." The downside is that any demonstrated benefits might be applicable only to a limited few who resembled the chosen subjects.

Growing concern about the restrictive nature of many efficacy or explanatory trials has led to interest in designing trials that take real-world considerations into account. An example of one of these *effectiveness*, or *management, trials* was performed by researchers from Seattle who were evaluating antidepressants.[1] Investigators were responding to the introduction of a new class of antidepressants known as serotonin reuptake inhibitors (SRIs) for treatment of depression. These new compounds had already been shown in explanatory trials to be beneficial in alleviating the symptoms of depression. They were also reported to have fewer side effects than traditional, tricyclic antidepressants and, thus, might make adherence to long-term treatment programs more feasible. The downside was that the drugs are considerably more expensive. The investigators designed the trial to answer the question, "Is initial treatment with a new SRI antidepressant, fluoxetine, better than initial treatment with either of two tricyclic drugs, desipramine or imipramine?" The "better" in this question encompassed several outcomes, including clinical improvement, quality of life, and economic considerations. The study was conducted in a large, staff model health maintenance organization in the Seattle area.

From the very start the researchers began breaking rules. They accepted into the trial virtually any adult patients who primary care physicians were intending to treat for depression. Exclusions were minimal. Only those with recent antidepressant drug treatment, alcoholism, or serious other mental disorders were kept from participation. Patients were admitted to the study regardless of medical comorbid conditions or severity of depression. Investigators then allocated subjects to 1 of the 3 drugs and broke the second golden rule. Neither physicians nor subjects were blind to the treatment assignment. This, the researchers argued, is as it is in the real world. Finally, if the two previous offenses were not enough to shatter the sanctity of the RCT, the researchers allowed subjects to change medications. That's right—real world.

Baseline measures of depression, anxiety, and quality of life were completed at baseline and periodically over a 6-month follow-up. Results are intriguing. There is evidence that the goal of enrolling a group of subjects typical of a primary care practice was achieved. Of the 621 patients referred by physicians for the study, 536 (86%) were actually randomized. That's a far cry from the 10–17% figures we have seen before. Depression and quality-of-life indicators improved comparably for all 3 medications over the 6 months of the study. However, the likelihood of continuing to take the initially assigned medication varied. Between 40 and 50% of patients assigned to desipramine and imipramine switched their medication to one of the other antidepressants (in most cases, fluoxetine) during the study. In contrast, only 20% of those initially assigned to fluoxetine changed. A major reason for this medication swapping was the occurrence of adverse effects. Within the first month of treatment, 27 and 28% of subjects assigned to the tricyclics discontinued these drugs because of adverse effects compared with only 9% for subjects assigned to fluoxetine. That is a big difference and confirmed what investigators suspected is a major cause of poor treatment success—not taking the medication.

When the economic aspects of the experiment were evaluated, medication costs for subjects assigned to fluoxetine were indeed higher than those experienced by patients assigned to the tricyclics; fluoxetine subjects' costs were twice as high. However, higher medication costs were offset by a tendency for fluoxetine-treated subjects to have fewer inpatient healthcare costs. The medication cost differentials between fluoxetine and the tricyclics were actually less than might have been anticipated. This result was due to the number of patients who began taking tricyclics and switched to the more costly fluoxetine. Because of the intention-to-treat analysis, these higher fluoxetine costs were attributed to the tricyclic group—as would occur in the real world. Overall, there was little difference in the total costs or clinical outcomes associated with initial prescribing of any of the 3 compounds.

Such results may be less than stunning. They are, however, useful. The research provides guidance to primary care physicians. It identifies differential rates of adverse effects for the medications under study, but suggests satisfactory outcomes for any of the 3 drugs so long as clinicians are alert to the possibility that close follow-up is required and a substitution of medications may be necessary. Even though several cardinal rules of randomized trials were ignored in this management approach, the findings have high external or real-world validity. We do need to remember, however, that with the lack of blinding of either subjects or referring physicians, reporting biases are possible. Widespread coverage of the "miraculous" benefits of fluoxetine at the time the study was conducted could easily have contributed to subjects' impressions of improved symptomatology. This is what occurs in the "real world." Therefore, in order for a management trial such as this to have validity, more rigorous, selective, carefully blinded, explanatory trials must be part of the overall evaluation.

Sometimes the value of an intervention lies exclusively in its practical application, including all the real-world impediments that this implies. Cisapride is a medication useful for treating heartburn due to gastroesophageal reflux disease. Serious safety concerns arose after the drug was found responsible for cardiac arrhythmias when given together with certain other medications.[2] In an attempt to alert Italian physicians of the dangers of coprescribing with cisapride, the health authority published a "Dear Dr" letter identifying the problem. To evaluate the effectiveness of this warning, a group of investigators carried out a time-series, cross-sectional study that examined prescriptions filled by the Italian National Health Service for time intervals before and after the warning letter. In the 2 years before the letter, 5.7% of cisapride prescriptions were coprescribed with contraindicated medications; in the 2-year after-period, the rate was 6.4%. The volume of cisapride prescriptions remained constant during the 4 years.

This seems a useful, if discouraging, finding. It suggests that, in the context of all the forces that come to bear on medical practice and prescribing, the advisory letter is insufficient to elicit change. Let us recall the design flaws imbedded in before-and-after methodology, however. Is it possible that there was some trend or concurrent cointervention that drove dangerous coprescribing up during the study interval and offset a beneficial effect of the letter? It seems unlikely. The results seem plausible after examining alternative hypotheses despite the known limitations of the study design. It is worth noting, however, that a time-series study, in which the result is negative (no change), is much easier to interpret than one that suggests success (coprescribing was seen to decline). An improvement in prescribing might be due to multiple other factors.

PRACTICAL CONSTRAINTS

Nonrandomized Interventions

When members of the Northern New England Cardiovascular Disease Study Group (NNECVDSG) wished to evaluate the effect of a 3-part intervention to improve hospital mortality following coronary artery bypass graft (CABG) surgery, they faced a practical problem.[3] The investigators knew that a randomized trial is the gold standard, but their situation was not well suited to the design. The group was relatively small, consisting of 5 hospitals with 23 surgeons who performed bypass procedures. Members of the group were to be the subjects of their own intervention. Random allocation and blinding are not easily accomplished in these circumstances. It is difficult to have a control group that is "unaware" of the intervention when researchers are also subjects. Therefore, the investigators used a before-and-after design.

The study was conducted over a 6-year period. Mortality data for CABG patients were collected from all 5 hospitals and included patients of all 23 surgeons. At the midpoint of the study, the intervention was begun. It consisted of distributing surgical outcome data to the participating doctors, conducting quality improvement training sessions, and making round-robin site visits to participants' programs to observe and share "best practices."

Figure 6–1 shows the pattern of mortality over time. The expected mortality rate was determined from a statistical model that predicted outcomes based on patient severity and other characteristics. An obvious decline from expected mortality is evident. The model predicted 308 deaths in the postintervention period. Instead, only 234 occurred—a 24% reduction. But recall the problems we have come to associate with before-and-after designs. How do we know that the decline in mortality is not due to changes in surgical risk of subjects over time or to some other, external secular events, such as a general improvement in surgical techniques?

The authors addressed these questions head-on. First, they compared characteristics of patients undergoing surgery in the 2 intervals to see if improved mortality was the result of operating on healthier, lower-risk patients. Researchers found that, in fact, postintervention subjects were older and had poorer cardiac function and more complicating, comorbid conditions—they were at higher rather than lower risk. Next, acknowledging that some turnover in participating surgeons during the 6-year study

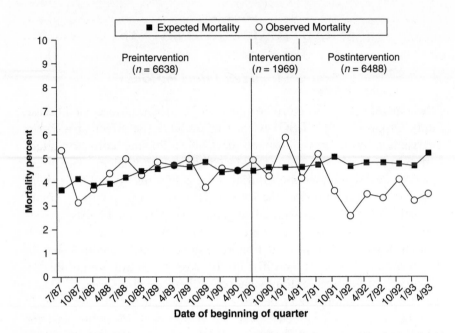

FIGURE 6–1. Expected and observed mortality for all patients (*n* = 15,095). The expected mortality is based on a risk model that includes age, sex, left main coronary artery stenosis, left ventricular ejection fraction, left ventricular diastolic pressure, and priority at surgery. (Modified, with permission, from O'Connor et al.[3])

was inevitable, researchers recognized that a change in the mix of surgeons might account for improvements. Perhaps younger, better-trained surgeons were replacing older, less skilled ones. They reran analyses, restricting results to include only subjects operated on by surgeons present during the entire study. Results were unchanged.

Throughout their discussion, the authors continued to examine competing explanations for the improved mortality rates. They considered the Hawthorne effect and acknowledged the possibility that external secular trends, such as improved technology, might have contributed to the improved outcomes. By comparing their results with national data, they determined that while nationwide mortality from CABG declined slightly (about 2.6% per year) during the study interval, the reduction was substantially less than that found in northern New England. All in all, this study is an impressive effort. When the ideal experimental design is not practical, the use of a "second-line" approach with a rigorous analysis may have to suffice. These authors acknowledged the shortcomings of their design but used methodological sophistication to make their results as plausible as possible.

A second example, which contains more than a dollar of irony, is the evaluation of the CONSORT guidelines for reporting on randomized trials.[4] Here, the question to be answered is whether implementation of the guidelines by medical journals accomplishes the improved methodological quality desired. The constraints are evident. The investigators who developed the intervention (the guidelines) were not in control of its implementation. This was up to the journals themselves. The researchers chose a sample of trials published in 4 widely read medical journals before guidelines were available and compared them with a second sample taken from the same journals after the guidelines were published. The quality of the published reports was assessed using the CONSORT checklist, as well as several other criteria related to methodological rigor.

Three of the 4 journals had adopted the CONSORT's guidelines; one had refrained. For the 3 adopters, the quality of reports showed a consistent improvement over the 2 time intervals. For the nonadopting "comparator" journal, slight but much less impressive improvements in quality were found. The researchers acknowledged the most critical limitation to their study design: that over the 4-year passage of time other events besides the guidelines might have contributed to the changes. The use of the nonadopting, comparator journal as an additional comparison certainly helps. Given the practical difficulties of mounting a randomized trial to evaluate this particular intervention, the before-and-after strategy may have to suffice.

Observational Approaches to Evaluating Efficacy

We tend to think of observational and experimental designs as different animals; the first identifies the risks of disease, the second evaluates interventions. The real distinction is not always clear. The risks that observational studies identify can be positive or negative—high cholesterol levels are bad but lowered cholesterol levels are good; diets low in fiber may lead to colon cancer, high-fiber diets are protective. Such observations lead quite naturally to treatment ideas. It is an easy step to infer therapeutic benefits from interventions that lower cholesterol levels or increase dietary fiber, even when data come from observational designs.

Observational methods are increasing in use as arbiters of treatment efficacy. There are reasons for this. Randomized clinical trials are expensive to mount, complicated to execute, and time consuming to complete. Sometimes a surgical procedure or medication has been modified or replaced before results of the "definitive" trial determining its efficacy are in. Observational designs, particularly the case-control and retrospective cohort approaches, are much more economical to perform and can often be accomplished before you can say "randomized double-blind controlled trial." As with the problem of evaluating mortality for CABG surgery that we have just explored, designing and executing randomized trials to evaluate some interventions is so complex that observational approaches seem quite appealing. We will examine several examples.

A. Cross-Sectional Ecologic: Many health interventions operate at a broad, societal level. These include laws, such as automobile seat belt requirements or cigarette advertising restrictions, or health service programs, such as organization of trauma services or provision of special dementia units for the elderly. While the interventions ultimately have an influence on individuals, it is their impact on groups that matters most and is often most amenable and appropriate for measurement. In these situations, a cross-sectional time-series approach using ecologic data is often seen. When one group of researchers wished to determine whether the passage of gun safety storage laws to protect children from unintentional injury from firearms could reduce mortality, their strategy was to compare rates of unintentional deaths from firearms in children before and after passage of a gun storage law.[5] They discovered that 12 states had passed such regulations between 1990 and 1994. These formed the basis for a time-series analysis. To adjust for secular trends in mortality across the country, national firearm mortality data between 1979 and 1994 were used. On the basis of national trends, expected rates for the 12 study states could be calculated by assuming that their rates would have mirrored those nationally in the absence of the laws. While rates of unintentional gunshot mortality declined during the interval from 1979 to 1994 on a national basis, the observed rates for the 12 study states fell an additional 23% after the passage of safe storage laws.

Recognizing that the time-series design is susceptible to problems arising from unmeasured cointerventions that occur at the same time as the study intervention, investigators were able to exert some control by accounting for secular changes in gun-related mortality in states without storage legislation. However, they still had the problem that within the study states other gun-control activities might be taking place. So, as responsible folks, they looked for ways to isolate the effects of the gun safe storage legislation. They noted, for example, that states that have enacted laws come from all regions in the country. These states do not appear to share characteristics such as demographic profiles that might explain the decline in mortality. Researchers also analyzed subcategories of gun-related mortality. They found that the *unintentional* gunshot death rate, which is the target of the laws, declined more than did suicide or homicide firearm mortality, the 2 categories of *intentional* injury being less likely to benefit from the legislation. Researchers also considered regression to the mean as an explanation for their findings. If the states where laws were passed had had particularly high rates of mortality compared with others across the country, regression (as was discussed in the last chapter) might have contributed to the decline. Prelegislation mortality rates were not higher in the study states, however.

Where does this leave the reader? The design is not perfect. Researchers have taken on an important question, but for reasons of practicality have resorted to an observational methodology; the design carries with it some important limitations. Yet they have done an admirable job of addressing competing explanations for the observed effect. It may not be a completely satisfying solution, but it may be as close as we are likely to get.

B. Follow-Up Design: The follow-up, or cohort, design is also used when controlled trials are difficult to implement. When investigators from Harvard wished to evaluate the potential benefit of physical activity on rates of heart attack and coronary heart disease death, they could have initiated an RCT. To do so would have been challenging, however. Although heart disease is the primary killer in the United States, measurable events, such as myocardial infarction and coronary death, are still infrequent enough that many subjects are needed to conduct a proper trial. Furthermore, exercise interventions require considerably more effort on the part of subjects who participate and investigators who monitor compliance than taking pills or performing procedures. Many people have difficulty adhering to an exercise protocol. Finally, a trial requires years of follow-up before a sufficient number of outcome events occurs. A more appealing option would be to take advantage of an ongoing cohort study that captured appropriate coronary event outcomes as well as data on exercise habits, had a large number of subjects enrolled, and was following up on them over a substantial period of time.

The Nurses Health Study turns out to fit that description perfectly.[6] Over 72,000 women who were in the age group 40–65 years when enrolled had the relevant data collected and had been followed up for 8 years. Recall that each nurse in the study completes a detailed health survey every 2 years. Included in the information reported are details on exercise and physical activity, such as walking, jogging, swimming, and bicycling. Details on medical outcomes, including coronary events, are also collected. By tabulating the number of physical activities that subjects report and converting them into standard energy expenditure units, known as metabolic equivalents, or METs, researchers were able to create a uniform measure of physical activity. One MET turns out to be the amount of energy expended per kilogram per hour by an individual at rest. The researchers calculated average weekly MET-hours for each subject and sorted subjects into 5 groups. As shown in Table 6–1, the lowest activity group averaged less than 1 MET hour per week, with the highest group averaging over 35 MET hours. The risk of coronary events *decreased* with *increasing* activity. (A relative risk of less than 1 indicates a benefit, or reduction in risk. A relative risk of 0.84 may be thought of as a 16% reduction in the likelihood of experiencing a coronary event; a relative risk of 0.68 indicates a 32% reduction.) Compared with the most sedentary group, increasing activity levels lowered heart attacks and coronary deaths by 23, 35, 46, and 54%, respectively. (The age-adjusted row under "relative risk" shows this.) Subjects in the second quintile with a relative risk of 0.77 have only 77% of the risk of events as those in quintile 1, for example. This means a reduction in risk of 23% (1.0–0.77).

An impressive result! But remember, this is an observational study, not a controlled trial. The design is "prospective"—data are collected before outcomes occur, and the quality of measurements and follow-up are excellent. Those items are positives. However, patients were not randomly assigned to exercise levels. They chose the type and the amount of activities themselves. Could this factor introduce bias? Could other risks for coronary outcomes travel together with exercise habits and be unevenly distributed among the groups? Absolutely. Table 6–1 shows this. Women who have higher levels of physical activity also smoke less and have lower body mass, less diabetes, and less high blood pressure. The study groups fail our experimental expectations that they are similar with respect to risks except for physical activity.

To deal with this unhappy situation, the researchers used *multivariable statistical modeling* techniques (we will discuss this topic later) to balance the groups—after the fact. These models adjust or account for a

TABLE 6-1

Distribution of indicators of coronary risk and outcomes
according to quintile group for total physical-activity
score at baseline and relative risk of coronary events

Variable	Quintile group for total physical activity[a]				
	1	2	3	4	5
No. of women	13,859	15,065	14,598	14,326	14,640
Total physical activity score (MET-hour/week)					
Median	0.8	3.2	7.7	15.4	35.4
	Percentage of group				
Risk indicator					
Currently smoking	28.2	23.7	19.6	17.4	17.5
History of hypertension	26.1	25.1	24.0	22.4	21.0
History of diabetes	4.2	3.3	3.7	2.8	2.6
History of hypercholesterolemia	12.0	11.4	11.7	11.6	10.6
Current postmenopausal hormone replacement therapy	19.5	21.5	23.1	23.8	24.1
Use of multivitamin supplement	36.9	39.9	43.0	45.0	47.2
	Mean				
Age, years	52.1	52.3	52.2	52.2	52.3
Alcohol consumption (g/day)	5.9	5.8	6.0	6.4	7.0
Body mass index	25.1	24.6	24.2	23.9	23.5
	Outcomes				
No. of coronary events	178	153	124	101	89
Person-year of follow-up	106,252	116,175	112,703	110,886	113,419
	Relative risk				
Type of analysis					
Age-adjusted	1.0	0.77	0.65	0.54	0.46
Multivariate[b]	1.0	0.88	0.81	0.74	0.66

[a]The total physical activity score was expressed as MET-hours per week, calculated as the average time per week spent in each of 8 activities; multiplied by the MET value of each activity. The MET value is the caloric needs during exercise divided by the caloric needs at rest.

[b]The model included variables for age (in 5-year categories), period during the study (four 2-year periods), smoking status (never smoked, previously smoked, or currently smokes 1-14, 15-24, or ≥25 cigarettes per day), body mass index (in 5 categories), menopausal status (premenopausal, postmenopausal without hormone replacement therapy, postmenopausal with previous hormone replacement therapy, or postmenopausal with current hormone replacement therapy), parental history with respect to myocardial infarction before the age of 60 years, multivitamin supplement use, vitamin E supplement use, alcohol consumption (0, 1-4, 5-14, or ≥15 g/day), history of hypertension, history of diabetes, history of hypercholesterolemia, and aspirin use (none, 1-6 doses per week, or 7 or more doses per week).

Modified, with permission, from Manson et al.[6]

variety of factors related to heart disease, including smoking, body mass, concurrent diseases, medications (including estrogens) and, of course, age. If these risks are present disproportionately in the groups with lower physical activity, they may share responsibility for outcome differences we are attributing to physical activity. One would expect that *adjusting* for these factors would blunt the apparent benefits of exercise. The lower rows of Table 6–1 indicate this is the case. The age-adjusted risks of coronary events across the exercise quintiles (multivariate analysis) are reduced, but they are still present and in the same order (0.88, 0.81, 0.74, and 0.66).

Figure 6–2 portrays graphically how the effects of physical activity are modified by factors such as smoking and body mass index. Note that when current smokers with the lowest level of physical activity are taken as the reference point (1.0), risk of a coronary event decreases as exercise increases, regardless of whether one is a current, previous, or never smoker. There is also a gradient of decreasing risk for any of the given activity levels by smoking status, with never smoking conferring the lowest risk (greatest benefit).

The approach taken by the Nurses Health Study investigators of thinking about a "risk factor" in terms of a positive behavior that could be promoted as an intervention makes perfect sense. Their use of an observational design as a surrogate for a clinical trial is becoming more common. The critical concern is, of course, the lack of unbiased allocation that one enjoys in a randomized trial. A critical assumption is that one can eliminate the potential bias created by subject or investigator selection by after-the-fact statistical adjustments. This seems a plausible approach so long as one is able to identify risk factors that may be unevenly distributed and lead to spurious findings. Multivariable statistical adjustments are only as good as the choice of variables used for adjustment. Sometimes authors employ only the most obvious characteristics, such as age and socioeconomic status. This approach will not be sufficient if other risk factors are left unaccounted for. Readers should check the "methods" to ascertain whether variables controlled for in the analysis seem appropriate and sufficient. In studies such as the Nurses Health Study, in which the population is large and a host of variables related to outcomes are collected, the chances for effective statistical adjustment are good. The concern always niggles, however, that some unmeasured forces are at play—associated with both physical activity and coronary events.

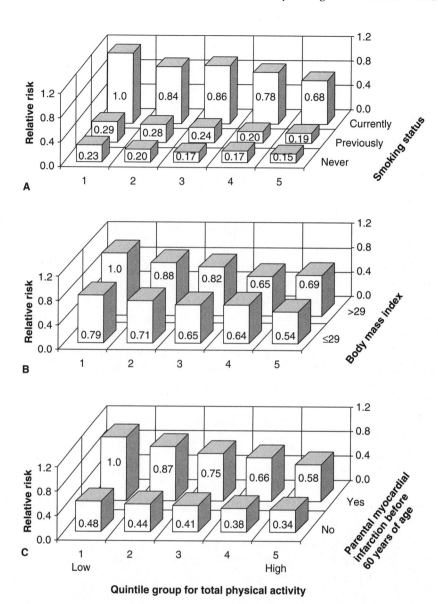

FIGURE 6–2. A: Multivariate relative risk of coronary events (nonfatal myocardial infarction or death from coronary causes) according to quintile group for total physical activity within subgroups defined according to smoking status. **B:** Body mass index, and **C:** Presence or absence of a parental history of premature myocardial infarction. For each risk factor, the reference group is the category at highest risk. Relative risks have been adjusted for the variables in the full multivariate model (listed in Table 6-1). (Modified, with permission, from Manson et al.[6])

ETHICAL CONCERNS

Sometimes the act of conducting a trial runs into ethical concerns. There may be strong feelings that investigators cannot withhold treatment for the control group. This situation can occur even when the intervention is not of proven value. Strong social pressures to approve a new cancer chemotherapy or AIDS antiviral agent can create a climate where RCTs are not feasible. Occasionally, an intervention will already be so entrenched in practice that pulling back to do a trial is unacceptable. Such is the case with Papanicolaou (Pap) smear screening programs to detect early stages of cervical cancer. A group of Canadian investigators were concerned that the efficacy of Pap screening programs had not been clearly demonstrated.[7] At the same time, they acknowledged the difficulty of carrying out an experimental study on a test that already enjoyed broad usage. They decided to conduct a case-control study, knowing that they were heading into selection bias problems as ". . . screened women tend to be of higher socioeconomic status than the unscreened and are thus less likely to get cervical cancer."[7]

Researchers identified 323 women with newly diagnosed invasive carcinoma of the cervix and obtained interviews on approximately two-thirds. They then sought 5 controls for each case, age matched within 10 years of controls, who also came from the same neighborhood and type of housing unit. The expectation was that matching would achieve socioeconomic comparability. Personal interviews were obtained by door-to-door canvassing. Although interviewers were not blinded to the hypothesis of the study, both cases and controls were told the investigation was a study of the "use by women of medical tests available in the community"; the mention of cancer was avoided. Among a battery of questions detailing personal and medical history were items related to obtaining a Pap smear as part of a routine, screening examination (as distinguished from one that was prompted by symptoms such as bleeding).

Results indicated that in the 5 years preceding the diagnosis of cancer, 32% of 212 cases had at least 1 screening Pap smear compared with 56% of the 1060 controls. This means that women who had not been screened were 2.7 times more likely to develop invasive cervical cancer than those who had. Screening appears to work. But what of the concerns over self-selection bias? Even though investigators had attempted to match cases and controls for socioeconomic status, they were concerned that this differential had not been eliminated and bias might still rear its unsightly head. Therefore, they subgrouped data according to categories of age, income, and educational attainment and performed a stratified analysis, as seen in Table 6–2. Examination of this table confirms that there are differential rates of Pap smear screening by age and the socioeconomic variables of income and education. Patients who were older and who had lower incomes and educational attainment were less likely to be screened. However, when one examines each stratum of age, income, or grade level achieved, the differential between frequency of Pap smears in cases and controls persists; the increased, *relative risk* ranges between 2.0 and 4.0.

Mindful of limitations of case-control studies, such as the representative nature of cases and controls, as well as other potential avenues for bias, the authors pushed their data further. They realized, for example, that they had not captured all the cases of invasive cervical cancer in their area. By working with the Provincial Cancer Registry, they found that

TABLE 6–2

Frequency of screening by Pap smear among cases and controls in relation to age, income, and education

	Frequency of Pap-smear screening		Relative risk
	Cases	**Controls**	
All subjects	67/212 (32%)	591/1060 (56%)	2.7
Age (years)			
20–34	7/16 (44%)	66/107 (62%)	2.1
35–44	18/36 (50%)	124/185 (67%)	2.0
45–59	31/102 (30%)	266/460 (58%)	3.1
60+	11/58 (19%)	134/304 (44%)	3.4
Total	67/212 (32%)	590/1056 (56%)	2.8
Income ($)			
<6000	9/45 (20%)	81/184 (44%)	3.1
6–9999	9/41 (22%)	65/124 (52%)	3.9
10–14,999	12/37 (32%)	128/217 (59%)	3.0
15,000+	16/35 (46%)	160/226 (71%)	2.9
Total	46/158 (29%)	434/751 (58%)	3.2
Highest grade achieved			
<9	22/78 (28%)	109/251 (43%)	2.0
9–11	19/64 (30%)	200/339 (59%)	3.4
12+	19/43 (44%)	214/328 (65%)	2.4
Total	60/185 (32%)	523/918 (57%)	2.5

Modified, with permission, from Clarke and Anderson.[7]

interviewed cases had Pap smear rates that were virtually the same as cancer cases who were not available for interview. So an unrepresentative collection of cases did not appear to be a problem. Selection of controls was also an issue. Almost 13,000 households were approached before the final sample of 1060 neighborhood controls was obtained. That is a success rate of only 1 in 12. Who was left out of the sample, and how did they differ from those who were selected? It turns out that about 8 of every failed recruitments was because no one was at home when the doorbell was rung. Other reasons include not finding a woman of the right age living in the household, inability of the woman to speak English, or refusal. To gain some estimate of the impact of this enrollment failure, the authors performed another subanalysis. They assessed screening rates in 232 controls who enrolled immediately after a case had been interviewed, that is, without an intervening failure. The rate of Pap smears was similar to that for the control group as a whole.

In a display of impressive tenacity, the investigators went on to explore other potential sources of bias, such as employment, access to medical care, smoking, interviewer bias, and selective recall. Their findings in each instance supported the benefits of screening. They found, for example, that while cases were more likely to be regularly employed, the relative risks associated with not being screened persisted when employed and not employed subgroups were analyzed separately. Recall bias was addressed by checking patient self-reports of Pap smears against medical records. Again, the benefits of screening held up.

The authors sum up their report with the modest conclusion that, "Although it may well now be too late to do a formal randomized trial of the efficacy of Pap smear screening . . . , we believe that this study has provided more convincing evidence in its favor than has previously been available."[7] One is inclined to agree. The investigators have addressed the challenges of the case-control methodology with vigor. It is difficult to think of many stones that have been unturned.

SUMMARY

Management, or real-world, trials can be useful adjuncts to explanatory efforts. They concede the tight control of the randomized trial in favor of assessing broader populations. They accept the realities of variable disease severity, concurrent diseases, inconsistent diagnostic criteria, adverse effects, and adherence problems. Within this context, methodological rigor can still prevail. Randomized allocation and intent-to-treat analyses are possible. Look for evidence that investigators have used whatever tricks remain to reduce possible bias and come up with plausible results.

When randomized trials are not practical, other experimental designs, such as the before-and-after or time-series, are often employed. These designs can suffer the ravages of secular trends. There may be activities occurring outside the experiment that influence results. Have authors identified these activities and attempted to control their effects? Have they compared risk characteristics of the before-and-after populations, or tried to use the same subjects to reduce variability? Have authors sought data from other sources to assess outcome trends external to the study?

Observational approaches to assessing efficacy are increasing. These are often prompted by the increasing costs and complexity of performing large-scale RCTs. Observational study designs are also used when trials are not feasible for practical or ethical reasons. These methods evoke all the concerns we have discussed in earlier chapters. Of overriding concern are selection biases that may create intervention and comparison groups that are dissimilar. If risks for the outcomes being measured are unevenly distributed, results may be tainted. Look for evidence that investigators have attempted to identify these risks and control their influence through stratified subanalyses or statistical adjustments.

Choosing the best design to study a problem is not always as easy as it first appears. Readers require some flexibility of mind and spirit. We must accept the reality that menus do not always meet our expectations. We should come to relish the challenges of some methodological variability and even inconsistency. This protects us from hobgoblins.

REFERENCES

1. Simon GE et al: Initial antidepressant choice in primary care: Effectiveness and cost of fluoxetine vs tricyclic antidepressants. JAMA 1996;275(24):1897.
2. Raschetti R et al: Time trends in the coprescribing of cisapride and contraindicated drugs in Umbria, Italy. JAMA 2001;285(14):1840.
3. O'Connor GT et al: A regional intervention to improve the hospital mortality associated with coronary artery bypass graft surgery: The Northern

New England Cardiovascular Disease Study Group. JAMA 1996; 275(11):841.

4. Moher D, Jones A, Lepage L: Use of the CONSORT statement and quality of reports of randomized trials: A comparative before and after evaluation. JAMA 2001;285:1992.

5. Cummings P et al: State gun safe storage laws and child mortality due to firearms. JAMA 1997;278(13):1084.

6. Manson JE et al: A prospective study of walking as compared with vigorous exercise in the prevention of coronary heart disease in women. N Engl J Med 1999;341(9):650.

7. Clarke EA, Anderson TW: Does screening by "Pap" smears help prevent cervical cancer? A case-control study. Lancet 1979;2(8132):1.

CHAPTER SEVEN

Making Measurements

I am giddy; expectation whirls me round.

TROILUS AND CRESSIDA, ACT III, SCENE II

W e have ruminated over study designs; tasted some problems, such as selective recall, loss to follow-up, and compliance bias; and sampled several solutions, such as matching, stratification, and random allocation. We are ready now to consider the implementation of these designs, that is, to examine how measurements are made and data acquired. After struggling with the complexities of study methodologies, gathering data would seem a straightforward proposition. By now it should come as no surprise that there are problems in this domain as well.

When measurements are made and data are collected, errors can occur. Children are improperly measured or their heights are incorrectly plotted on the growth curve; a Pap smear is not correctly read; items on a personality-inventory scale are left blank or filled in incorrectly. The list of unfortunate possibilities is almost endless, and the chance that data acquired by researchers do not properly measure the attributes they wish to determine is a potent hazard. Although errors in data collection can occur anywhere in the process—from obtaining the measurements through entering data for computer analysis—we will focus on problems that occur at the interface between subjects and investigators. It is here that the most serious errors occur and the only point at which readers have a shot at detecting difficulties. We will discuss two general types of errors, those that occur in an unpredictable fashion and those that are made in a biased, systematic way.

RELIABILITY & VALIDITY

Two terms that readers will encounter whenever measurements are mentioned are *validity* and *reliability*. We have already discussed the concept of validity as it applies to the overall acceptance of study results, whether conclusions are justified based on design and interpretation or, in the case of external validity, whether results can be generalized to settings and subjects outside those described in the study. As used to describe data, *validity* refers to the degree to which a measurement represents a true value, such as how closely a blood pressure determination represents a subject's true blood pressure or a depression questionnaire captures a person's true mental state. *Reliability* relates to the reproducibility of measurements. How closely do repeated measurements on the same subject agree? Both these attributes are important to clinical studies and are related. Errors can be caused by a lack of either validity or reliability. If 6 students attempt to measure a patient's blood pressure and obtain values that range from 110/70 to 145/95 mmHg, the results lack reliability. This creative group of estimates may be due to changes in the patient's anxiety level, differences in inflation of the cuff, or variable auditory acuity among the students. The results also lack validity. Better reproducibility is necessary to achieve a valid result but does not guarantee it. If a cuff of the wrong size is employed or the manometer is out of calibration, each of our 6 students might come up with a blood pressure reading of 145/95 mmHg, a totally reliable finding that does not represent the true pressure.

VARIABILITY OF THE UNSYSTEMATIC SORT

Over recent years, we have come to appreciate an amazing spectrum of variability that occurs when health researchers attempt to make measurements. Problems of reliability pervade every aspect of the work, from history taking and the physical examination to laboratory and x-ray investigations to survey completion. In part, the problem is due to subject variation. Pulse rates and blood pressures may change from one observation to the next. A subject who swears he never eats carrots when completing a dietary recall admits a passion for all sorts of vegetables on personal interview. Human frailties on the part of observers also contribute. Examiners become fatigued, are inattentive, or simply have not been trained to make measurements in a standardized manner. Regardless of the underlying reason, observers assessing the same subject, the same symptom, the same skin rash, or the same diet frequently come up with differing interpretations.

In a study by Derryberry on "the reliability of medical judgments on malnutrition,"[1] 6 pediatricians were asked to independently examine one hundred and eight 11-year-old boys and rate their nutritional status. Each boy was examined by each physician and rated on a 4-point scale that ranged from "excellent" to "poor." In the author's understated prose, "the results of this investigation were disconcerting." Ratings of the 6 physicians showed marked variation. One physician rated 15 of the 108 boys as having poor nutritional status; another rated only 2 in that category. Twenty-five different boys were given the "poor" rating by at least 1 of the doctors, and only 1 child received a unanimous judgment of poor by the entire group of evaluators. Two youngsters received every rating from excellent through poor in the course of the 6 evaluations.

Elements of the physical examination that would pretend to high objectivity are subject to observer variability. Meade et al reported on differences among 3 physicians of "comparable clinical experience" who were given the task of palpating the peripheral pulses of 84 hospitalized patients.[2] For this experiment, the examiners had only to record whether a particular pulse was present or absent. To spice up the game, 12 of the patients were recycled through the examination so that they were evaluated twice by each of the 3 observers. Table 7–1 summarizes some of the findings from this study. Agreement ranged from as high as 97% for palpation of femoral pulses to as low as 69% for the dorsalis pedis pulse. If this interobserver problem were not bad enough, results from the 12 patients who underwent a second pulse check highlighted further deficiencies. Intraobserver error, that is, a rater's change from a previous assessment, also occurred. When the 3 examiners were checked on the 48 pulses that they assessed on 2 occasions, they changed their minds about the presence or absence of a pulse from 13 to 27% of the time.

The pronouncements of those who interpret the technological trappings of medicine are not immune from the problems of observer variation. Lack of agreement among experts reading coronary angiograms,

TABLE 7-1
Agreement of 3 observers examining femoral, posterior tibial, and dorsalis pedis pulses in 96 male patients (192 observations)

	Agreement, all present	Disagreement, present/absent	Agreement, all absent	Percent total agreement
Femoral	187	5	0	97
Posterior tibial	126	40	26	79
Dorsalis pedis	105	59	28	69

Modified, with permission, from Meade et al.[2]

electrocardiograms, and radiographs has been demonstrated. Variability of this sort affects research studies as well. A study that attempted to document recognition rates of osteoporosis-related vertebral fracture among older hospitalized women offers an example.[3] The goal of this research was to determine how frequently clinicians were aware of the presence of vertebral fractures that were evident on routinely obtained lateral chest radiographs on patients who had been admitted to the hospital for other reasons. Two experienced radiologists reviewed a sample of 934 lateral chest films to determine how many demonstrated fractures of the thoracic spine. Definitions of fracture were provided to each radiologist from published guidelines. When the radiologists were asked to identify fractures that were moderate to severe, agreement was not good. One radiologist found an overall prevalence of 15.6%; the other indicated that 28.5% of patients had fractures. When only severe deformities were considered, agreement was better, 8.0 and 8.7%, respectively. Where does the truth lie in this situation? How many patients actually had vertebral fracture? The researchers resolved their dilemma by accepting only fractures where both radiologists agreed one was present. That left a prevalence of 14.1%—probably an overly conservative estimate of the true frequency.

Even assessments we revere as "gold standards" are susceptible. In an exercise related to a multicenter trial exploring the effects of beta-carotene on cervical dysplasia, 4 pathologists were asked to examine and grade 106 biopsy specimens.[4] Each slide was reviewed by each pathologist, who rated the specimens as belonging in 1 of 5 categories of dysplasia: (1) none, (2) mild, (3) moderate, (4) severe, and (5) carcinoma in situ (CIS). Variability for the readings of the 106 slides may be seen in Table 7–2.

TABLE 7-2

Percentage agreement of 4 pathologists' classification of cervical dysplasia on 106 slides (comparison with "index" pathologist)

Grade of dysplasia, "index" pathologist	Grade of dysplasia, 3 pathologists				
	None	Mild	Moderate	Severe	CIS
None	**35**	47	12	6	0
Mild	7	**54**	30	8	1
Moderate	1	21	**50**	26	2
Severe	1	7	35	**49**	8
CIS	0	6	19	54	**22**

CIS, carcinoma in situ.
Modified, with permission, from DeVet et al.[4]

The table shows the percentage of agreement when the first pathologist's readings are compared to those of the other 3 pathologists. The bold numbers (running diagonally) represent complete agreement, with cells furthest from the diagonal representing the greatest discord—a bit of tarnish to be sure.

Most of the errors we have been discussing occur in a haphazard or unpredictable fashion. They can be troublesome, since without reasonable measurement reliability, the validity of study results will be compromised. However, minor, random variations tend to even out—some higher and some lower—and, human imperfection being what it is, can never be entirely eliminated.

SYSTEMATIC ERROR

There are, however, more dangerous brands of error. These occur when variations in measurements take on a predictable or biased aspect. An example comes from a study devised to determine the accuracy of clinical measurements of fetal heart rates.[5] In this investigation, an electronic fetal monitor was attached to record the intrauterine heart rate. At the same time, members of the hospital staff counted the heartbeats by auscultation. Observer variations in the range of 20% of the monitored rate were discovered. However, the pattern of this variability did not occur randomly. Fetal heart rate is a guide to the infant's well-being. A rate in the neighborhood of 130–150 beats/min suggests that labor is progressing satisfactorily. Heart rates that fall below 130 or rise above 150 suggest that problems may be brewing and that the fetus is experiencing distress. Figure 7–1 depicts the patterns of observer variation that occurred with

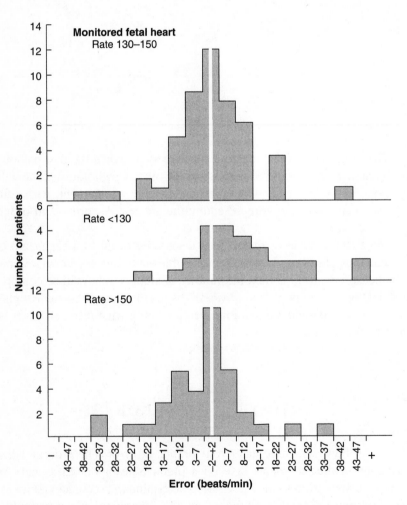

FIGURE 7–1. Error of auscultation of hospital staff at different fetal heart rates. (Modified, with permission, from Day, Maddern, and Wood.[5])

differing monitored fetal heart rates. When the true rate is within the 130–150 range, observer errors appear evenly scattered between overestimates and underestimates; but if monitored rates rise or fall to levels that indicate distress, the pattern of errors no longer appears symmetrically distributed. When the monitored rate drops below 130, observer errors tend to overestimate the rate, that is, bring it back toward the desirable range. When the rate exceeds 150, there is a tendency for observers to make estimates on the lower side of the electronic value.

This situation represents biased error. The cause for the bias is understandable; the hospital staff is not looking for trouble. They want healthy deliveries and babies with good outcomes. Nevertheless, the message is clear. As with poor, giddy Troilus, expectation plays tricks on the mind. The wishes of the observer can influence measurements. Opportunities for measurement bias are abundant in medical studies and are one more problem that journal readers need to sniff out.

Investigator & Interviewer Biases

Measurement biases can be produced on both sides of the investigator-subject dyad. For those who are collecting information for a study, the pitfalls are numerous. One's investment in the results or anticipation of how subjects are likely to respond can easily become a self-fulfilling prophecy. This is not to impugn the integrity of investigators. Objectivity is difficult to master. It is difficult for surgeons not to find benefits from their favorite operative procedures to alleviate hemorrhoids or for social workers—looking for evidence of abuse and neglect—not to uncover child maltreatment in a group known to be at high risk. It is unfair to expect an investigator trying a new antihypertensive agent to display total disinterest when taking the blood pressure of a subject under treatment. Even when investigators are not directly involved in data gathering, difficulties can occur. Choi and Comstock evaluated the effect that the personalities of hired interviewers had on subject responses to questionnaires in a community mental health survey.[6] The instrument, administered by 6 different interviewers, measured a variety of mental health characteristics, including sensitive items like troubles with alcohol, suicidal thoughts, nervous breakdowns, and stressful life events. In checking for observer variation, the authors noted that interviewer C produced subject scores that differed substantially from those of her colleagues. When the investigators attempted to identify items in the questionnaire that interviewers found embarrassing, interviewer C reported feeling uncomfortable with questions pertaining to suicide, menstruation, marital happiness, and personal habits; none of the other 5 interviewers seemed disturbed by these topics. The authors concluded that a measurement bias was operating—that the personality and beliefs of the particular interviewer were systematically affecting responses on her questionnaires.

Subject Biases

Subjects can also introduce bias into the data-collection process. When subjects are invested in the experiment, have ideas about which therapy might be preferred, or simply want to please investigators by responding in a favorable way, results may be altered. Patients who believe that a certain method of childbirth is beneficial are likely to report high satisfaction and favorable outcomes for their infants; parents of hyperactive children who have become convinced that food additives cause their child's aberrant behavior will see improvement in symptoms when these presumed toxins are eliminated from the diet. Most patients want things to be better. They want to do things right! In fact, there is such a tendency for subjects to wish to respond in what they perceive as a correct fashion that the term *social desirability bias* has been coined to describe the phenomenon.

Subjects are often reluctant to admit to habits they know are damaging to their health. Researchers who have investigated the association between passive smoking (exposure to secondhand cigarette smoke) frequently use nonsmoking spouses of smokers as subjects for these studies. When these spouses have increased rates of lung cancer compared to unexposed controls, the accusing finger points to the secondhand smoke. The worry has been, however, that social desirability bias, a reluctance to confess to the bad habit of smoking, may have influenced some spouses to underreport their own smoking habits. If many of these subjects are classified as nonsmokers when, in fact, they smoke, study findings could be biased. Passive smoking could be blamed for diseases brought on by primary, direct exposure to cigarettes.

To assess this potential bias, researchers combined results of several studies that compared self-reports of smoking status with individuals' blood levels of cotinine, a major nicotine metabolite.[7] Modest levels of cotinine may appear in the blood of passive smokers, but more substantial levels are possible only in active smokers. Finding high cotinine levels in subjects who report "never smoking" constitutes misclassification. Table 7–3 shows

TABLE 7–3
Misclassification rates for current smokers self-reported as either never smokers or former smokers (in percent)

	Self-reported smoking status			
	Never smokers		Former smokers	
	Occasional[a]	Regular[a]	Occasional[a]	Regular[a]
Majority females	6.0	0.8	9.8	0.7
U.S. minority females	15.3	2.8	5.6	2.3
Majority males	5.1	1.4	7.1	2.3
U.S. minority males	19.7	3.7	13.2	3.3

[a]True smoking status based on cotinine level.
Modified, with permission, from Wells et al.[7]

the percentage of those who claim "never a smoker" status reclassified by cotinine levels. These results indicate that a number of subjects who claim innocence are smokers. The authors conclude that social desirability is occurring, that it varies by racial group and that, while present, is probably of insufficient magnitude to create the association between passive smoking and disease.

Another source of consternation for investigators trying to observe subjects and collect data on them is that the act of observation may change the behavior. This phenomenon goes under the fancy name of the *Hawthorne effect* (named not for a person but for a manufacturing plant where the effect was observed). The essence of the problem is that people may act differently when they know they are being watched. Examples of particular interest to clinicians come from projects that attempt to alter physician behavior, such as studies that try to improve the way doctors order laboratory tests or prescribe medications. Generally these efforts aim at educating physicians and stressing logical approaches to better decision making. Beneficial effects demonstrated in these experiments may as often be due to the Hawthorne effect as to planned edification, however. Evidence to support this suspicion is found in the typical pattern that physician behavior follows in the wake of interventions. Inappropriate test ordering or prescribing generally decreases for a time, creating a satisfaction in the investigators that comes from watching rational enlightenment. Delight is usually short lived, however. Given a few additional months, behavior reverts to its previous wayward level, suggesting that the transient improvement was related to the presence of the study rather than its message.

The report of an evaluation of an educational program to reduce ordering of thyroid function panels demonstrates this rebound phenomenon.[8] Here the authors attempted to influence physicians' laboratory utilization during an educational conference in which doctors could characterize and analyze their motives for test ordering. In the 3-month period following the conference, the ordering of thyroid function panels dropped (see Figure 7–2). However, as time went on and clinicians forgot either about what they had learned or about the dark shadow of the investigators hovering over their shoulders, rates returned toward preintervention levels.

In the course of studies on practitioner-patient interactions, Starfield and colleagues found evidence that presence of an observer in the room with the doctor and patient changes the practitioner's recognition of patient problems.[9] When medical records completed after visits that were observed were compared with those of visits where no observer was present,

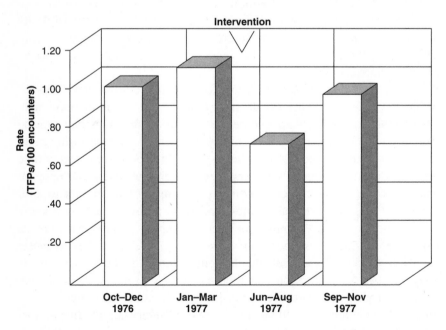

FIGURE 7–2. Rate of ordering thyroid function panels (TFPs) by 3-month quarters. (Modified, with permission, from Rhyne and Gehlbach.[8])

it was found that a significantly higher percentage of patients' previous concerns were noted when the observer was in attendance.

Increasing comfort or familiarity with the measuring devices used to collect data may also affect subject response. It has been noted, for example, that patients having their blood pressures measured for the first time are much more likely to have elevated readings than after they have become acclimated to the medical setting. Studies that utilize pretests and posttests to measure knowledge or repeat administrations of psychological inventories run the risk that a subject's earlier experience with the instrument will modify scores of subsequent administrations. Pretests may give learning clues or provide test-taking experience that makes the posttest easier; subjects may remember their previous responses to questions in a psychological battery and be influenced by these when they are retested later.

All this means that investigators must be extremely cautious not to influence the course of human behavior in the process of observing it. For the reader, the lesson is to be on guard for biases introduced by the process of making measurements and to look for evidence that authors have taken steps to minimize the errors of data collection.

REDUCING MEASUREMENT ERROR

There are several steps researchers can take to deal with the problems of unreliable and biased measurements. Some of them are already familiar. Keeping observers and subjects *blind* is probably the best-known technique for reducing bias. In the *double-blind* trial, neither the investigator nor the subject is allowed to become aware of which particular intervention is being used for any given subject. This approach is particularly suited for drug trials, where identical pink capsules can be concocted to contain the placebo and the active drug. There are some obvious limitations. It is very difficult, for example, to conceal the queen-sized bed and rococo decor of a birthing room from either physicians or patients. When measurements are made of interventions where investigators cannot maintain ignorance of the allocation, independent observers from outside should be brought in. In the Leboyer childbirth study described in Chapter 5, for example, outcome assessments of neonates were made by observers who were kept scrupulously unaware of the method of childbirth used to bring the baby into the world.[10]

There are other techniques for improving measurement reliability and minimizing observer error. These include establishing unambiguous standards, validating instruments, providing observers with supervised training and practice, and using multiple observers or data sources.

Establishing Unambiguous Standards

When all observers are clear on exactly how measurements are to be made, variability is reduced. Agreement on what size blood-pressure cuff should be used for which size arm and whether the fourth or fifth Korotkoff sound should be used as the diastolic estimate will produce more reliable blood-pressure measurements. Deciding in advance how many millimeters an ST segment must be elevated to be compatible with an infarction pattern on an electrocardiogram will improve the consistency of the diagnosis of heart attack. Researchers who work on the vertebral fracture problem have convened and published a set of guidelines to standardize the determination of fractures.[11] Measurement devices should, of course, be standardized and calibrated. Questionnaires should be pretested and unclear or ambiguous items deleted or revised.

Validating Instruments

Investigators who study the benefits of physical activity on health often depend on subjects' self-reports to derive their estimates of energy expenditure. Typical survey instruments employ the strategy of asking subjects to estimate the average time they spend each week engaged in various sorts of physical activity, such as working or jogging, bicycling or swimming, walking or climbing flights of stairs. Investigators can employ several strategies to assess their accuracy. These methods include testing the reproducibility of responses by administering instruments to the same groups over different intervals of time and by comparing results with those obtained from other instruments that attempt to measure the same variables. Readers should recognize these approaches as attempts to assess reliability (reproducibility) and validity, respectively.

The Nurses Health Study relies extensively on subjects' self-reports. A portion of their extensive questionnaire asks subjects to report on the frequency with which they engaged in a set of common physical activities during the course of a year. The investigators selected a small subset of their large cohort who had completed this activity questionnaire and asked them to complete a series of weekly activity diaries and past-week recall assessments over the course of a following year.[12] Reporting past-week recalls of activity offered improved accuracy by offering a much smaller time frame for subjects to remember activities. The diaries required participants to log their activities on an hourly basis and so provided a highly detailed comparison. At the end of the year, subjects were asked to complete another activity survey like the first.

Such an approach has both value and limitations. It is useful to discover how closely subjects' responses to the same instrument will compare over time and how more detailed assessments of activity compare with broadly stated annual averages. Investigators in the Nurses Health Study found that in their sample both the reproducibility of responses after a year (reliability) and agreement between the broad annual and more intensive estimates of activity correlated reasonably well. There was variation, however, and as a system to test the performance of the questionnaire, there are limitations. The "validating" instruments are still relying on self-reporting, and there is an underlying assumption that subjects' activities remain unchanged over the 1-year interval. Such may not be the case.

When another group of researchers wondered about the validity of their physical activity questionnaire, they used another approach.[13] After subjects in this study had completed a short self-administered questionnaire on physical activity, each was outfitted with an electric pedometer, a small instrument attached to the waist that measures each stride a person takes. Pedometers were worn for 7 days. Because researchers were interested in validated self-reported daily walking, the pedometers were removed when participants engaged in sports or recreational activity.

Comparisons of self- and electronically reported walking were illuminating. Both men and women substantially underreported the average distance they walked each day. In fact, the questionnaire captured only one-third of the walking distance documented by the pedometers. This means that any research estimates of energy expenditure based on the questionnaire are significantly below the mark and hints that a redesign of the questionnaire is in order.

Providing Observers with Supervised Training & Practice

Once the guidelines for measurements have been established, observers need to practice their interviewing skills or measuring techniques to see where variations or biases are likely to occur. Training need not be extensive or elaborate to improve measurement validity. As part of a national study of the relationship between colon polyps and cancer, a proficiency testing program was begun to monitor the accuracy of interpretation of fecal occult blood tests.[14] Eight coordinators from clinical centers were tested with preprepared stool samples before a 1-hour instructional seminar, immediately after the seminar, and several months later. Instruction focused on the proper addition of reagents and correct interpretation of color changes for the test. Findings are presented in Table 7–4.

Overall, the percentage of slides read correctly increased from 60% for the preintervention period to 91% in each of the postintervention periods. Most of this improvement was seen for the intermediate, "moderately positive" samples.

Using Multiple Observers or Data Sources

Although we have recognized the problems that multiple observers have in agreeing with one another, several opinions are usually better than one. It is good form, for example, when diagnostic studies such as radiographs or pathology specimens are involved in results, to send these bits of gold to independent observers for a second opinion. Even projects that rely on data acquired through seemingly straightforward methods such as chart audits are better served when information is checked by more than one observer. Use of multiple sources of data is another useful technique for improving validity. Recall from Chapter 3 that Ross et al[15] used medical and pharmacy records to verify the estrogen use reported by subjects, and

TABLE 7–4

Percentage of correctly interpreted Hemoccult tests before, immediately after, and several months after training

Reading	Before	Immediately after	Months after
Strongly positive	78	97	100
Moderately positive	38	90	94
Negative	94	81	86

Modified, with permission, from Fleisher et al.[14]

Wynder and Graham performed a special substudy to demonstrate that the reported smoking habits of cases and controls were not influenced by investigator bias.[16]

Knowledgeable researchers will assess interrater reliability and supply readers with estimates of how closely different raters agree. The information is usually offered in terms of percent agreement or a correlation coefficient, with higher values signifying better reliability. Better still are reports that provide estimates of agreement that have taken chance into account. When the 4 pathologists sort cervical cytology slides into 5 categories, chance alone dictates that there will be some concordant groupings.[4] The study investigators reported agreement as a kappa value, a statistic that adjusts their findings to account for this chance agreement. Kappa values range between 0 and 1.0. Values above 0.6 are generally required to indicate acceptable agreement. In the vertebral fracture study, the kappa for radiologist's agreement on moderate and severe fractures was only 0.56; agreement for severe fractures was a healthier 0.80.[3]

While there are few guarantees that a research article is free from measurement error, readers may derive some comfort from evidence that authors have been rigorous in the pursuit of objective data. As with investigators who demonstrate cognizance of study-design problems, authors who set forth the methods they use to guard against measurement error are more likely to gain our confidence.

SUMMARY

When measurements are made, errors will occur. Pay particular attention to whether authors have done the following:

1. Attempted to improve reliability by (a) establishing unambiguous measurement standards, (b) subjecting instruments to test-retest or validating comparisons, (c) utilizing trained observers, and (d) corroborating observations.

2. Taken steps to guard against biased measurement. Where possible, are both subjects and investigators blind to subject allocation? If the identity of treatments cannot be concealed, are attempts made to incorporate independent observers who are unaware of study hypotheses or treatment allocations?

REFERENCES

1. Derryberry M: Reliability of medical judgments on malnutrition. Public Health Rep 1938;53:263.
2. Meade TW et al: Observer variability in recording the peripheral pulses. Br Heart J 1968;30:661.
3. Gehlbach SH et al: Recognition of vertebral fracture in a clinical setting. Osteoporos Int 2000;11(7):577.
4. DeVet HCW et al: Interobserver variation in histopathological grading of cervical dysplasia. J Clin Epidemiol 1990;43:1395.
5. Day E, Maddern L, Wood C: Auscultation of foetal heart rate: An assessment of its error and significance. Br Med J 1968;4:422.
6. Choi I, Comstock GW: Interviewer effect on responses to a questionnaire relating to mood. Am J Epidemiol 1975;101:84.
7. Wells AJ et al: Misclassification rates for current smokers misclassified as nonsmokers. Am J Public Health 1998;88(10):1503.
8. Rhyne RL, Gehlbach SH: Effects of educational feedback strategy on physician utilization of thyroid function panels. J Fam Pract 1979;8:1003.
9. Starfield B et al: Presence of observers at patient-practitioner interactions: Impact on coordination of care and methodologic implications. Am J Public Health 1979;69:1021.
10. Nelson NM et al: A randomized clinical trial of the Leboyer approach to childbirth. N Engl J Med 1980;302:655.
11. National Osteoporosis Foundation Working Group on Vertebral Fractures. Assessing vertebral fractures. J Bone Miner Res 1995;10(4):518.
12. Wolf AM et al: Reproducibility and validity of a self-administered physical activity questionnaire. Int J Epidemiol 1994;23(5):991.
13. Bassett DR Jr, Cureton AL, Ainsworth BE: Measurement of daily walking distance-questionnaire versus pedometer. Med Sci Sports Exerc 2000;32 (5):1018.
14. Fleisher M et al: Accuracy of fecal occult blood test interpretation. Ann Intern Med 1991;114:875.
15. Ross RK et al: A case-control study of menopausal estrogen therapy and breast cancer. JAMA 1980;243:1635.
16. Wynder EL, Graham EA: Tobacco smoking as a possible etiologic factor in bronchiogenic carcinoma: A study of six hundred and eighty-four proved cases. JAMA 1950;143:329.

CHAPTER EIGHT

Analysis: Statistical Significance

There are three kinds of lies: lies, damn lies, and statistics.

DISRAELI

$\mathbf{M}$r. Disraeli's discomfort with statistics is shared by many. Somehow the brief exposure to the courses offered in college or medical school seems woefully inadequate. A working understanding of P values, chi-squares, and the null hypothesis is difficult to come by and easily lost. The current sophistication of statistical presentations in journal articles makes it tempting to abdicate responsibility for interpretations of statistical significance to statisticians and editors, but that is probably not a wise plan.

For the most part, statistics and clinical research work well together. Testing for statistical significance keeps overly optimistic clinical anecdotes in a proper perspective, but there are instances where the fit is not good and the clinical message of the study is drowned in a statistical flood. In this chapter, we will explore the principles underlying the use of tests of statistical significance, clarify some statistical terminology, and look at some common, subtle (and usually unintentional) statistical traps that await the unwary reader.

INFERENCE

To understand statistical significance, we need to know about making inferences. An *inference* is a generalization made about a large group or population from the study of a sample of that population. To illustrate, suppose you have just completed Saturday morning house calls and stopped by Pritchard's country store to take in a Dr Pepper and some rural wisdom. Behind the flour sack on which you perch are two apple barrels: one holds red Jonathans, the other, Golden Delicious (to which you are partial). Unfortunately, there has been some mixing of the two varieties, so the red apple barrel has some goldens in it and vice versa. Proprietor Pritchard, always keen for a wager, says he will give you your favorite if you correctly identify the red-apple and golden-apple barrels by examining only 5 apples. You reach back, extract the apples from one of the barrels and, finding that 1 is red and 4 are yellow, announce that you have found the golden-apple barrel.

You've just made an inferential statement, that is, a judgment about a characteristic of a population (the composition of a whole barrel of apples) from evaluating a sample of the population (5 apples). Simple enough. However, there is a chance that you are wrong. The proportions of your sample may not reflect the composition of the entire barrel. You may have chanced to pick the only 4 yellow apples in the entire red-apple barrel, made an incorrect inference, and lost the bet. To reduce the likelihood of making an error, your best strategy would be to enlarge the size of your sample. Instead of 5 apples, you could examine 20; or you could increase your sample to 50 or 100 apples. As you come closer to counting the entire barrel of apples, your chance of making a mistaken inference decreases. If, finally, you study all the apples, you are no longer making an inference, and you can be certain of the composition of the barrel.

Most medical studies, whether testing the efficacy of steroids in treating poison ivy dermatitis or looking for an association between exposure to asbestos and occurrence of lung tumors, evaluate samples of larger populations. We examine 50 patients, 200 workers in a single industrial plant, or even an entire community, hoping to generalize about all patients, all chemical plants, or society at large; and as with picking apples at the country store, there is a chance that we will be misled by our sample.

SAMPLING VARIABILITY

Let us suppose we are interested in testing a claim that the antibiotic azithromycin causes less diarrhea than amoxicillin/clavulanate. We begin by giving azithromycin to 50 patients in our practice. We ask the patients to report any episodes of diarrhea that occur while they are taking the medication. It turns out that 6 patients (12%) report diarrhea. So far, so good. We would like to be able to predict the behavior of all patients who receive azithromycin. To verify our earlier results, we select another sample of 50 patients and repeat the experiment. This time only 8% of patients experience the side effect. Repeating the experiment yet a third time reveals an incidence of diarrhea of 10%.

In attempting to delineate the true incidence of diarrhea for all patients who receive the drug, making inferences from samples of 50, we have uncovered the problem of sampling variability. Each estimate we gather is at slight variance from its predecessor. If we continue repeating our samples of 50 patients, we will find that our collection of results begins to form a pattern. Values begin to cluster around certain recurrent percentages. The results group around 10%, which is not only the most common result (the *mode*) but is located in the center of the distribution (the *median*). We find some estimates both higher and lower than 10%, but these become less frequent as they become more extreme.

If we had nothing better to do than continue taking our samples of 50 patients over and over, we would form a sampling distribution for the incidence of diarrhea among people given azithromycin. Figure 8–1 illustrates what this distribution might look like. The conclusion we draw from examining the distribution is that the true incidence of this side effect is about 10%, with the understanding that any estimate we make from a single sample of 50 patients may be slightly off the mark. We can examine the plot of diarrhea frequencies and estimate how often we would find a rate as high as 16% or as low as 4%. Assuming that our experiments are performed reliably, we can predict that this will occur relatively infrequently—about 1 in 20 times.

We still have not answered the question of whether azithromycin has a lower frequency of diarrhea associated with its use than does amoxicillin/clavulanate. Let us find another group of 50 patients, subject them to amoxicillin/clavulanate treatment, and ask for reports of diarrhea. The patients provide us with the information that 16% of them encountered the side effect. That is an apparent increase over the 10% figure we calculated

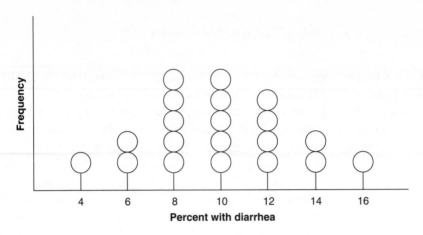

FIGURE 8–1. Percentage of patients receiving azithromycin who develop diarrhea. Based on 20 samples of 50 patients each.

for azithromycin, but we did note that, occasionally, sampling variability would produce an estimate as high as 16% for the frequency of azithromycin-induced diarrhea. Does the rate we have found for our single sample of amoxicillin/clavulanate patients represent a true difference from azithromycin, or have we drawn the 1-in-20 sample from the high end of the same distribution?

THE NULL HYPOTHESIS & STATISTICAL SIGNIFICANCE

To help answer the question, we need to invoke a major nemesis—the *null hypothesis.* Lack of understanding of just how the null hypothesis operates causes countless headaches. It is different from a research hypothesis. The proposition that azithromycin causes less diarrhea than amoxicillin/clavulanate is a research hypothesis. We expect that by comparing the 2 drugs, we will find a difference in the incidence of this side effect. The null hypothesis states that there is no difference to be found between the items being compared—in this instance, the 2 drugs. The null hypothesis is strictly a statistical convention, used for helping us decide how likely it is that our results have been produced by quirks of sampling.

Testing for statistical significance using the null hypothesis has been likened to the judicial process of assuming innocence until guilt is proven. We make the assumption (contrary to our research hypothesis) that the true incidence of diarrhea for the 2 preparations is no different: amoxicillin/clavulanate is innocent of causing more diarrhea. Taking on the role of prosecuting attorney, we then try to demonstrate beyond reasonable doubt that in fact there is a difference. Rejecting the null hypothesis supports the research hypothesis.

We know that repeating the azithromycin experiment on 50 people would yield a result of 16% incidence of diarrhea only 1 in 20 times. That is a reasonably unlikely occurrence. So when we learn that amoxicillin/clavulanate causes diarrhea in 16% of patients in our single sample, we have useful evidence to argue. We can say that if amoxicillin/clavulanate really behaved like azithromycin, it would be unlikely (a 5% chance) that we would find a 16% or higher rate of diarrhea in a single sample. This 5% probability is referred to as the *P value*. It is the likelihood of obtaining a result this extreme if the null hypothesis were true. We feel that a 1-in-20 chance is too small to continue to support the null hypothesis, so we reject it and proclaim that our findings are "statistically significant": the drugs cause diarrhea at different rates.

Most often, results of clinical studies are said to be statistically significant, that is, unlikely to be due to chance, if the *P* value is less than 5% (.05) or 1% (.01). But there is nothing magical about these levels of probability. The .05 tradition began in the 1920s with an influential statistician named Fisher. It has been habit ever since. Frequently we read articles in which a wide variety of *P* values is used, ranging from .05 to values that are many times smaller. Small *P* values like .001 or .0001 are important to the extent that they tell us that differences we observe are unlikely to be mistakes in inference due to sampling, but we need to be wary of a subtle illusion that is created by these impressive numbers.

SOME PROBLEMS OF STATISTICAL SIGNIFICANCE

The Size of the P Value Does Not Indicate the Importance of the Result

It is tempting to believe that very small *P* values indicate great discoveries. Terms such as "highly significant results" and "very highly significant results" are liberally sprinkled through journals. Consider an article that demonstrated a correlation between alcohol consumption and elevated blood pressure.[1] In this study, the amount of daily intake of alcoholic beverages was compared with blood pressure readings for patients in a prepaid group practice. A difference in average blood pressure was found between individuals who drank small amounts of alcohol and those with high intake. Those who drank more had higher blood pressure. This finding was reported as statistically significant, with a P value of 10^{24}. Extraordinary! Enough "highlys" in that significant result to cover an entire page. But what does this value really mean? Simply that the difference found is not likely to have occurred because of sampling alone. It does not mean that the findings are of major medical importance, nor does it mean that alcohol consumption is a major cause of hypertension. It means only that chance is an unlikely explanation for the results. This extremely small P value is due to the size of the sample, 80,000 people in all. Very large samples become close approximations of the populations they are estimating, so any differences that are found are likely to be real (like examining all the apples in the barrel). There is little reason to report such an extreme P value. The results are scarcely more credible than had they been achieved with a value of 1 in 10,000. Yet it is difficult for a reader not to be awed by such a statistical tour de force, even though it adds nothing of substance to the study.

Results May Be Statistically Significant but Practically Unimportant

Just as it is easy to be impressed by small P values, so can we be seduced into equating statistical significance with clinical or practical importance. To learn more about the outcome of primary care residency training programs, a group of investigators tracked career choice, board certification, and practice location for groups of internal medicine and pediatrics residency graduates.[2] Comparisons were made between doctors trained in "traditional" and "primary care" programs. One finding that was featured in the abstract of the report was that "board certification rates in internal medicine were statistically higher for graduates of primary care training programs (80%) than for graduates of traditional programs (76%, $P = .002$) but were not statistically significant for both groups of pediatric graduates."[2] Here, another small P value seems portentous. But how important are these results? Table 8–1 elaborates on the data.

TABLE 8–1

Percentage of graduates of internal medicine and pediatrics training programs who are board-certified

	Percent certified, number of graduates	
	Internal medicine[a]	Pediatrics[b]
Traditional training	76 (12,594)	80 (3411)
Primary care training	80 (1156)	76 (772)

[a]Difference between traditional and primary care training statistically significant ($P = .002$).
[b]Difference between traditional and primary care training not statistically significant ($P = .089$)
Modified, with permission, from Noble et al.[2]

It turns out that the 80 to 76% differential in certification rates found among internal medicine graduates is exactly reversed for pediatricians. Eighty percent of traditional program graduates are certified, compared with 76% of those from the primary care residency. Why should the same percentage-point difference prompt a significant P value for internists while leaving pediatricians out? Three times as many internists were included in this study as pediatricians, and sheer force of numbers enabled the authors to reject the null hypothesis in one instance but not in the other. In fact, the small difference in certification rates is of little importance. In discussing results, the authors even point to the group *similarities* as evidence of comparable preparation from the training tracks. Somewhere along the way, the glint of the significant P value proved too alluring, and a statistically significant but practically questionable result became a prominent part of the report.

A large Finnish trial testing the effects of two vitamins with antioxidant properties on the development of angina pectoris provides another illustration of P value problems.[3] Over 22,000 male smokers 50–69 years of age were randomly allocated to receive either alpha tocopherol (vitamin E) or beta-carotene in a 2×2 factorial design. This is the same design used by the Physicians' Health Study. It allows the assessment of two interventions in a single effort. In the current example, the 22,000 Finns were allocated to 1 of 4 groups with about 5500 subjects in each. Every subject took 2 pills daily—one group took both vitamins, another took alpha tocopherol and a placebo, a third, beta-carotene placebo, and the fourth, 2 placebo capsules.

Each year subjects were interviewed by trained nurses to determine the number of new cases of angina that had developed. After 7 years, angina had developed in 1983 subjects. Fewer of these were in the group taking alpha tocopherol than in the placebo group. The P value of this statistical comparison was .04. That is less than the .05 required to reject the null hypothesis and looks like a positive result. Alpha tocopherol prevents angina. But the P value does not tell the entire story. It says little about the magnitude or importance of the result.

The reduction in new angina cases due to taking alpha tocopherol was only 9%. Researchers followed up on their subjects for a total of 96,000 person-years (every subject in the study for 1 year contributes one person-year). When angina rates are compared, those taking alpha tocopherol had 19.6 new cases of angina per 1000 person-years compared with 21.5 per 1000 for those not taking the vitamin (see Table 8–2). The difference, less than 2 cases per 1000 person-years, is not large. The question can be asked, "Is a benefit of this size clinically important?" Is widespread deployment of alpha tocopherol advisable given this magnitude of effect?

Further inspection of Table 8-2 might raise eyebrows higher still. Beta-carotene users developed angina at a higher rate than placebo recipients. There were 21.2 new cases per 1000 person-years of observation compared

TABLE 8–2

Incidence of angina pectoris after supplementation with either alpha tocopherol or beta-carotene for Finnish men (n = 22,269) followed up for 4.7 years on average

Supplementation	Number of cases	Incidence per 1000 person-years[a]	P value	Difference[b] (95% confidence interval)
Alpha tocopherol	948	19.6	.04	−9% (−17% to −1%)
No alpha tocopherol	1035	21.5		
Beta-carotene	1020	21.2	.19	+6% (−3% to + 16%)
No beta-carotene	963	20.0		

[a]1 person-year accumulates for each year a subject remains under observation.
[b]Comparison between angina incidence for those taking and those not taking the supplement.
Modified, with permission, from Rapola et al.[3]

with 20.0. However, this result is not statistically significant. The P value was calculated at .19. The observed difference could have occurred by chance according to the convention of using $P < .05$ as the dividing line. There is not much difference between the two comparisons—a 9% reduction in angina for alpha tocopherol compared with a 6% increase in angina for beta-carotene. Yet one finding is stamped as "statistically significant," while the other is not.

Differences That Are Not Statistically Significant Are Not Necessarily Unimportant

We have already agreed that most medical researchers look for differences and that rejecting the null hypothesis "proves" the difference. However, failure to reject the null hypothesis does not guarantee that differences observed are not real or that the results being compared are the same.

In the Physicians' Health Study there were almost twice as many heart attacks among placebo recipients as among doctors who took aspirin—239 versus 139 with approximately 11,000 doctors in each group.[4] The P value associated with this difference is less than .00001. That means the result is most unlikely to be a chance occurrence. There is little disagreement with the statistical or practical importance of the finding. When the investigators moved to examine the effect of aspirin on stroke, however, some less agreeable information emerges. Among aspirin takers there were 119 strokes compared with only 98 among placebo recipients. As seen in Table 8–3, this finding was not statistically significant. The P value was .15, meaning that a difference like this or more extreme could have occurred 15 out of 100 times the experiment was repeated. This is too often to reject the null hypothesis. But let's look further.

There are several pathogenic mechanisms that cause strokes—ischemia and hemorrhage. As aspirin inhibits platelet aggregation, one might expect it would exert a beneficial effect in protecting subjects from ischemic stroke while exacerbating the likelihood of bleeding. The researchers did a subanalysis (Table 8–3) that depicts stroke outcomes according to the two categories. There is little difference between aspirin and placebo recipients (about a 10% increase in ischemic strokes for aspirin takers), and the P value reflects this. However, hemorrhagic stroke occurs almost twice as often in the aspirin group (23 cases versus 12 in the placebo group). The P value of this finding "just misses" the mark of statistical

<table>
<tr><td colspan="5" align="center">**TABLE 8−3**</td></tr>
<tr><td colspan="5" align="center">**Cardiovascular outcomes in the aspirin component of the Physicians' Health Study according to treatment**</td></tr>
</table>

End point	Aspirin group	Placebo group[a]	P value[b]	Relative risk[b] (95% confidence interval)
Myocardial infarction	139	239	.00001	.56 (.45-.70)
Stroke	119	98	.15	1.22 (.93-1.60)
Ischemic	91	82	.5	1.11 (.82-1.50)
Hemorrhagic	23	12	.06	2.14 (.96-4.77)
Unknown cause	5	4	-	-

[a]Over 54,000 person-years of observation were made for each group.
[b]Of end point for aspirin group compared with placebo. Risk below 1.0 is protective; above 1.0 is harmful.
Modified, with permission, from Steering Committee of the Physicians' Health Study Research Group.[4]

significance at .06. Does this mean that aspirin does not place patients at increased risk for hemorrhagic stroke? Not at all. It simply means that for the number of episodes of stroke and magnitude of difference observed, we are unable to reject the possibility that the difference was due to chance. But we are left with considerable discomfort that this "not statistically significant" finding may be clinically important. One stroke more in the aspirin group or one less among placebo recipients, and we might have had a P value that broke the .05 barrier.

BETA ERRORS & STATISTICAL POWER

Two kinds of mistakes can be made in the search for statistical significance. The first occurs when we reject the null hypothesis and it is true. We claim that two treatments are dissimilar and, in fact, they are no different. This is an alpha, or type I, error and occurs when we claim different rates of diarrhea for amoxicillin/clavulanate and azithromycin when, in fact, the drugs behave no differently. The second potential hypothesis-testing error is suggested in the case of aspirin and strokes. Failing to reject the null hypothesis when it is not true is a beta, or type II, mistake. A true treatment effect or difference is being overlooked. Table 8–4 schematizes the correct and incorrect decisions that can be reached when we are testing the null hypothesis. Rejecting the notion that two treatments are identical when they are different and finding no difference when none exists are correct decisions. Of the incorrect conclusions, the alpha error is most familiar to clinicians. We worry about claiming that a new treatment is effective when chance could have produced the difference we observe. We are accustomed to seeing P values, and conceptualization of this first type of error is reasonably straightforward.

Coming to an understanding of beta errors is a bit trickier. We wish to avoid making the mistake of missing a therapeutic or causal effect; that is, of accepting the idea that two treatments are the same simply because we cannot reject the null hypothesis and state that they are different. However, once we start speaking of rejecting and accepting differences, the question becomes, "Differences of what size?" The range of possibilities is infinite. When we contemplate the likelihood of missing a treatment effect in our hypothesis testing, the size of the difference we are looking for is crucial. For each possible difference that might exist, there is a different probability of making a beta error. The whole business of beta error is an interplay between the magnitude of difference, the number of subjects involved, and the alpha level at which experimenters decide they will reject the null hypothesis.

TABLE 8–4

Errors encountered in testing the null hypothesis to evaluate efficacy of treatments A and B

		Null hypothesis (treatment A = treatment B)	
		True (no difference)	**False** (difference)
Decision (based on statistical test)	**Accept** (No difference)	Correct	Type II, beta error
	Reject (Difference)	Type I, alpha error	Correct

Researchers can lessen their chances of making beta errors by altering these 3 basic ingredients. We speak of the process of reducing beta error as improving experimental power. Statistical power is the complement of beta error (power = 1 − beta error); the lower the beta error, the greater the power. The power of an experiment is the likelihood that the experiment will detect a treatment effect of a particular size (a difference) for a particular number of experimental subjects. The higher the power, the better our chances of finding the treatment benefit, if it is there. The most obvious way of increasing power is to increase the number of subjects studied. Power is also influenced by the size of the difference between groups. For a given number of subjects, an experiment will have a higher probability of detecting a large treatment effect than a small difference. Power may also be improved if we are willing to raise the alpha level. But to increase the likelihood of finding a statistically significant difference by changing alpha, we must also increase the possibility of falsely claiming an experiment effect. Comfort with these concepts requires some pondering, but they are worth trying to master. Several discussions of the topic are available.[5-7]

Ideally, power calculations should be made before an experiment is performed. Investigators should decide on the number of subjects they require on the basis of estimates of the size of the difference they wish to detect and the certainty with which they desire to pinpoint that difference. In general, a power of 80-90% is considered respectable. However, things do not always work out that way.

Freiman and colleagues analyzed 71 studies from major medical journals that reported negative results; that is, no difference was found between treatments studied.[7] The investigators found that a high percentage of these studies could have missed an important difference in therapies because an inadequate number of subjects were evaluated. Many of the studies actually showed trends suggesting that a treatment worked, but the authors concluded that the therapy was no different from control simply because they could not reject the null hypothesis. Results reported in experimental and observational studies may be negative not because there are no differences but because the power of the study was too low to detect meaningful differences. Researchers should comment about power when they present negative results. They should provide some estimate of the probability that, for the number of subjects studied and the alpha level considered reasonable for rejecting the null hypothesis, a meaningful difference between groups would have been detected. Presenting confidence intervals is also of help.

CONFIDENCE INTERVALS

Many now feel that the confidence interval (CI) gives readers more useful information than the *P* value alone. The value of *P* provides a standardized estimate of the likelihood that we would encounter differences as large as or larger than those we have discovered if there were actually no difference or effect (the null hypothesis were true). But we do not learn anything about the size of the result itself. When CI reporting is used, a point estimate of the result is given together with a range of values that are also consistent with the data at hand. When this range is large, many possible results must be considered—some much greater than the estimate provided by the study, some much smaller. Sometimes the CI includes zero difference between two therapies or no risk associated with an exposure, and we must concede that corticosteroids may not benefit meningitis patients or caffeine intake lead to heart attack.

Confidence intervals give us a more intelligent reading of the results of the studies on vitamin supplements and angina and the Physicians' Health Study than *P* values alone. In the vitamin/angina study, subjects taking alpha tocopherol had a statistically significant (*P* = .04) reduction in new onset of chest pain (see Table 8–2). Those taking beta-carotene were "no different" from placebo takers (*P* = .19). One treatment worked; one did not. But the point estimates and CIs provide a subtler interpretation (see Table 8–2). Alpha tocopherol takers had a 9% lower incidence of angina; that is the point estimate. However, the study results were consistent with angina reduction of as much as 17% or as little as 1% (the 95% CI). Beta-carotene, on the other hand, is estimated to increase angina by 6%, with results consistent with an *increase* of as much as 16% or a *decrease* of 3%. In the alpha tocopherol arm of the trial, the confidence interval does not include 0 (no effect); in the beta-carotene arm, it does. But the range of the CI for the two vitamins is very similar, albeit in opposite directions. The study authors are alert to this nuance when they conclude, "We found evidence of a preventive effect of alpha tocopherol supplementation on angina pectoris, but the effect was small and hardly of public health significance. Beta-carotene supplementation had no preventive effect; in fact, a slight increase in the incidence of angina pectoris was observed."[3]

Interpreting results of the aspirin arm of the Physicians' Health Study also needs more than *P* values alone can provide. Table 8–3 indicates that aspirin reduces heart attacks by 44% (the point estimate) and that findings are compatible with a benefit that may be as high as 54% or as low as 30%. This is helpful information; it gives a good sense of the practical importance of results. But now look at the point estimate and CI for hemorrhagic stroke. Here an increase of over 100% was found, a result that could be plausibly as high as 300%. Of course, the data are also compatible with a decrease of 4% and, as the CI includes 0, no difference at all. This is the reason that the investigators were unable to reject the null hypothesis. When a 95% CI contains 0 difference, it is equivalent to saying that one is unable to reject a no hypothesis at the 5% level. Recall that the P value for hemorrhagic stroke was .06. Wide CIs indicate greater uncertainty about the true value of a result; a small CI narrows the reasonable choices. But, as the hemorrhagic stroke findings indicate, the greater information provided by CIs makes the simple P value, "reject or don't reject" approach seem less than fully informative. Several journals have published useful discussions about CIs,[8–11] including their use to assess clinical and statistical significance at the same time.[12]

Alternative Explanations of the Observed Difference

Having observed differences that are statistically significant, we are tempted to conclude that our treatments or theories are responsible for observed effects. Unfortunately, this may not be true. Remember, when we reject the null hypothesis, we only assess the role chance may have played in creating differences.

Capricious methodology may still be at play. Biases, such as the subject-allocation bias seen in the birthing-room experiment[13] or the selective recall of the nurses with multiple sclerosis,[14] could be responsible for results. When important methodological flaws occur, statistical proclamations become superfluous. The British statistician Sir Austin Bradford Hill has remarked that too often "the glitter of the t-table diverts attention from the inadequacies of the fare."[15]

SUMMARY

Statistical tests need to be kept in proper perspective. Tests of significance tell us about the role that sampling variability may have played in results. They make no other claim on the validity of the study. All our concerns about the effects of sampling procedures, proper measurement, and the many opportunities for bias still pertain. Readers who can keep their heads when those about them are lost in a swirl of *P* values have an advantage. They can concentrate on issues of relevance.

Ask the following questions:

1. Are the differences observed between the groups under study likely to be due to chance?

2. If differences are not due to chance, do they occur because of biases, or are they related to the treatment or another study factor?

3. If differences are statistically significant (not due to chance), are they practically important?

4. If differences are not statistically significant, is it possible that a true difference has been overlooked (a type II error made)?

REFERENCES

1. Klatsky AL et al: Alcohol consumption and blood pressure. N Engl J Med 1977;296:1194.
2. Noble J et al: Career differences between primary care and traditional trainees in internal medicine and pediatrics. Ann Intern Med 1992;116:482.
3. Rapola JM et al: Effect of vitamin E and beta carotene on the incidence of angina pectoris: A randomized, double-blind, controlled trial. JAMA 1996;275(9):693.
4. Final report on the aspirin component of the ongoing Physicians' Health Study: Steering Committee of the Physicians' Health Study Research Group. N Engl J Med 1989;321(3):129.
5. Sterne JA, Smith GD: Sifting the evidence—what's wrong with significance tests? BMJ 2001;322(7280):226.
6. Berwick DM: Experimental power: The other side of the coin. Pediatrics 1980;65:1043.
7. Freiman JA et al: The importance of beta, the type II error and sample size in the design and interpretation of the randomized control trial: Survey of 71 "negative" trials. N Engl J Med 1978;299:690, 694.
8. Bulpitt CJ: Confidence intervals. Lancet 1987;1:494.
9. Confidence intervals extract clinically useful information from data, editorial. Ann Intern Med 1988;108:296.

10. Gardner MJ, Altman DG: Confidence intervals rather than P values: Estimation rather than hypothesis testing. BMJ 1986;292:746.
11. Rothman KJ: A show of confidence. N Engl J Med 1978;299:1362.
12. Braitman LE: Confidence intervals assess both clinical significance and statistical significance. Ann Intern Med 1991;114:515.
13. Goodlin RC: Low-risk obstetric care for low-risk mothers. Lancet 1980;1:1017.
14. Ascherio A et al: Hepatitis B vaccination and the risk of multiple sclerosis. N Engl J Med 2001;344(5):327.
15. Hill AB: The environment and disease: Association or causation? Proc Roy Soc Med 1965;58:295.

CHAPTER NINE

Analysis: Some Statistical Tests

A student set forth on a quest,
To learn which of the world's beers was best,
But his wallet was dried out
At the first pub he tried out,
With two samples he flunked the means test.

The type of statistical maneuver an author chooses depends on properties of the data that need to be analyzed, how the data are distributed, and what questions they are to answer. Statisticians speak of 4 types of data: nominal, ordinal, interval, and ratio. *Nominal data* are, as the appellation implies, named categories. ABO blood groups, male or female sex, and treatment cures or failures are examples. These data have no mathematical relationship to one another; they are neither ranked nor ordered. Sometimes numbers or letters are used to identify categories, such as license plate numbers, numbers on baseball uniforms, or designations such as diabetes type 1 or type 2. Although these numbers may be convenient as identifying symbols, it must be remembered that they are only symbols with no mathematical properties. They cannot legitimately be added or subtracted from one another. From an analytical point of view, each is a separate entity having an equivalent weight or value.

Ordinal data can be sequenced or ranked—smallest to largest, lightest to heaviest, easiest to most difficult, "always agree" to "never agree." Examples include socioeconomic classes, military grades, academic ranks, medical conditions (such as stable to critical), or health-status indicators (such as excellent, good, fair, and poor). These represent ranks, but the distances or intervals between the categories are not necessarily uniform. It is clear to almost everyone that excellent health is preferred to good health and that good health is better than "fair" or "poor" health. But how much better is excellent than good? Is the difference between good health and fair health the same as the difference between fair health and poor health? One cannot say. The order is understood, but the intervals between classes are not defined and cannot be assumed to be equivalent.

That claim can only be made for *interval* and *ratio data*. These data share the properties of having rank or order, but they also have known, equal distances between values. Ratio data have a true zero point as well as equal intervals, but this distinction is not a major sticking point for most of the statistical testing encountered in our reading. We will speak of interval and ratio data together as *continuous* data. Temperature, height, weight, and blood sugar concentration share the properties of equal intervals. The distance between 33°C and 34°C is the same as that from 39°C to 40°C. The loss of 2 g of hemoglobin is the same, whether the level drops from 16 to 14 g or from 10 to 8 g (even though the clinical implications may not be the same).

Continuous data lend themselves readily to arithmetic operations such as addition and subtraction, and if there is a true zero in the interval scale (kilograms, inches, hematocrit), multiplication and division are possible. Data of this sort can be averaged to give the mean height for eighth-grade girls from Spokane or the mean blood lead level for workers in a battery warehouse.

Nominal and ordinal data must be handled more gingerly. Because they are categorical and lack mathematical equivalence, they cannot legitimately be added or subtracted. Different types of statistical tests are appropriate.

To make the world of statistical tests a bit less foreign, let us look at some examples of several of the most commonly used statistical approaches to analyzing medical data. The objective here is not to become proficient in performing these tests but to gain an intuitive feel for how the data are being handled. For those who need a more detailed understanding, several statistics texts are available, and general-readership journals periodically publish helpful articles on statistical topics.

Let us suppose that we are conducting an experiment to find a remedy for the many patients who complain of fatigue. Over the years, we have noted that several remedies appear useful, but we have never subjected them to the close scrutiny that our increasingly critical sensibilities tell us is required. Two treatments come to mind: Lydia Pinkham's Compound

TABLE 9 – 1

Condition of patients after receiving Lydia Pinkham's Compound or Bull Durham's Extract—observed values

| Treatment | No. of patients | | | Total |
	Much peppier	Somewhat peppier	Not improved	
Lydia Pinkham's	14	19	9	42
Bull Durham's	9	11	18	38
Total	23	30	27	80

and Bull Durham's Liver Extract. Accordingly, we approach the next 80 patients who visit with the chief complaint of "feeling tired" and ask them to participate in our study. All willingly agree to be randomly allocated to one of the two treatments. They consent to swallow a teaspoonful of either Lydia Pinkham's Compound or Bull Durham's Liver Extract 3 times a day for the next 2 weeks. Naturally, we have made certain that the 2 tonics look and taste the same and that the bottles are labeled with a study number to which only a pharmacist friend has the identifying key. After patients have completed the full course of treatment, we quiz them about any change in level of energy, classifying each into 1 of 3 categories: much peppier, somewhat peppier, or not improved.

Of the 80 patients we enroll, 42 are randomized to the Lydia Pinkham group and 38 are dosed with Bull Durham. Patient outcomes are seen in Table 9–1. Inspection of the table suggests that more patients improved with Lydia Pinkham's than with Bull Durham's, but some patients in each group are much improved and some failed to improve at all. Is Lydia Pinkham's superior to Bull Durham's in relieving fatigue?

TESTS FOR CATEGORICAL DATA

The test most commonly used for these categorical kinds of data is called the *chi-square test*. The chi-square statistic takes the distribution of results (much peppier, somewhat peppier, and not improved) for the two samples (Lydia Pinkham's and Bull Durham's) and gives us an estimate of the likelihood that these two samples are representative of the overall population. What is the distribution of all fatigued people who report their state of energy 2 weeks after a course of medication? Are our 2 treatment distributions different enough from one another that they are not likely to have been drawn from the same parent population? Are the differences we observe real or simply an artifact of sampling variability?

To answer this question, we need some notion of the "true" population values. Our best approximation from the data at hand is the number of patients in each category from the total number of subjects in our study—the combined sample of patients given Lydia Pinkham's and Bull Durham's. These figures are seen in the lowest row of Table 9–1, the "bottom marginal." Among all our patients, 23 reported feeling much peppier, 30 were somewhat peppier, and 27 remained unimproved. The chi-square test uses these marginal values as an estimate of the population, or as *expected values* if no differences existed between the treatment groups. The *observed* number of cases in each cell is compared with the number that would be expected on the basis of the distribution of the bottom marginal. Each expected value is calculated by multiplying the total number of patients in each treatment group by the proportion of each outcome represented in the bottom row of each column (Table 9–2). The difference between each observed and expected value is squared, divided by the particular expected value, and summed to give the value of chi-square. This number is matched with a standard table of chi-square values to determine the probability that the collection of observed and expected differences could be explained by chance. The larger the difference between what we observe and what we expect, the larger the value of chi-square and the lower the P value. Table 9–2 shows how a chi-square statistic would be calculated for our experiment. The summed value of 6.09 would occur only 5 in 100 times by chance ($P = .049$), so, according to common practice, we could reject the null hypothesis that the Lydia Pinkham's and Bull Durham's treatments were no different, that is, that the figures are estimates of the same population. We then conclude that since we believe our experimental design to have avoided biases that could account for the observed treatment responses, Lydia Pinkham's does a better job than Bull Durham's at pepping up our patients.

There are other statistical tests that take advantage of the ordered sequences of categorical data. The outcomes of our Lydia Pinkham–Bull

TABLE 9-2

Condition of patients after receiving Lydia Pinkham's Compound or Bull Durham's Extract—expected values

	Category			
Treatment	Much peppier	Somewhat peppier	Not improved	Total
Lydia Pinkham's	$42 \times {}^{23}\!/_{80} = 12.1$	$42 \times {}^{30}\!/_{80} = 15.7$	$42 \times {}^{27}\!/_{80} = 14.2$	42
Bull Durham's	$38 \times {}^{23}\!/_{80} = 10.9$	$38 \times {}^{30}\!/_{80} = 14.3$	$38 \times {}^{27}\!/_{80} = 12.8$	38
	23	30	27	80

$$\text{chi-square} = \text{sum of} \frac{(\text{observed} - \text{expected})^2}{\text{expected}}$$

$$= \frac{(14-12.1)^2}{12.1} + \frac{(19-15.7)^2}{15.7} + \frac{(9-14.2)^2}{14.2} + \frac{(9-10.9)^2}{10.9} + \frac{(11-14.3)^2}{14.3} + \frac{(18-12.8)^2}{12.8}$$

$$= 0.30 + 0.69 + 1.90 + 0.33 + 0.76 + 2.11$$
$$= 6.09, P = .049$$

Durham experiment (much peppier, somewhat peppier, and not improved) are ordinal data. However, when we employed the chi-square test, we really treated them as if they were nominal data (equal in value) only; we failed to incorporate the additional information that "much peppier" is better than "somewhat peppier," which is better than "not improved." By failing to take advantage of this useful information, we lost efficiency or power in our statistical testing. We used a lower-octane test when a higher-octane test was available and appropriate. In so doing, we jeopardized our ability to detect a difference between our two treatments when one was indeed present—the type II error we discussed in the previous chapter. Although in this situation chi-square was sufficient to detect a difference in our treatment groups, a shift in the categories of only one or two patients might have lowered the value of chi-square, giving us a slightly higher P value, and we would not have rejected the null hypothesis. Selecting a more powerful test reduces that risk.

TESTS FOR CONTINUOUS DATA

Other statistical maneuvers are available to medical researchers that can legitimately be used only on continuous data under conditions in which the data can be assumed to be normally distributed. The most commonly encountered is the *t* test, or Student's *t*, named not because of the delight the procedure evokes among students struggling with statistics but in honor of the British mathematician who developed it. This man's name, as it turns out, was Gossett, and he worked not for any of the prestigious medical research units of Great Britain but for the Guinness Brewery. Guinness employed Gossett to work out statistical sampling techniques that would improve the quality and reproducibility of its beer-making procedures. Gossett published his statistical work under the name of "Student," presumably to keep his trade secrets from the eyes of Guinness competitors.

Student's *t* test compares the means of two samples of observations to help the researcher (or brewer) decide whether the samples are likely to come from the same or different populations. Anytime continuous data are collected on two groups of subjects, you are likely to find *t* tests being used. Differences between the blood pressures of patients eating high- and low-sodium diets, or examination scores for students given self-instruction programs instead of lectures, or lengths of hospital stay by patients enrolled in fee-for-service or prepaid insurance programs all can be assessed by using *t* tests. To construct and interpret a *t* test, one needs to know the size of the samples, the magnitude of differences between the two sample means, and the variability of the data in each sample. When the difference between two means is large, the variability among data is small, and the sample size is reasonably large, the likelihood is increased that the sample means represent two different populations. The summary *t* statistic and its corresponding calculated *P* value can be used as a guide for rejecting the null hypothesis.

To illustrate, let us return to our fatigue experiment. We have a hunch that improvements in fatigue found in our patients who took Lydia Pinkham's Compound have a physiologic basis. We suspect that many of our tired patients in fact have anemia. The magic of Lydia Pinkham's, we hypothesize, is due to its iron content, which raises the hemoglobin level of patients and is responsible for their increased pep. Accordingly, we obtain hemoglobin determinations on patients in both treatment groups at the completion of therapy. The resulting distributions of hemoglobin levels for the Lydia Pinkham's and Bull Durham's patients are displayed in Figure 9–1. As can be seen from this visual display, the group of Lydia Pinkham's patients appears to have a greater number of higher hemoglobin values. If we calculate posttreatment mean hemoglobin levels for each group by summing the observations and dividing by the total number of subjects, we find that Lydia Pinkham's subjects' average hemoglobin value is 13.6 g, compared with 12.6 g for the Bull Durham's patients. Does this difference of 1 g between the means indicate that the samples represent different populations and that patients who plied themselves with Lydia Pinkham's and reported feeling better have higher levels of

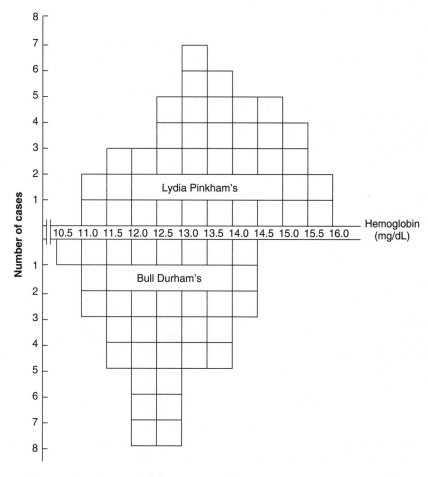

FIGURE 9–1. Hemoglobin levels of patients treated with Lydia Pinkham's Compound and Bull Durham's Extract.

hemoglobin? Or is the difference simply due to sampling variability? The *t* test helps answer this question.

For the 42 patients who received Lydia Pinkham's Compound, the average posttreatment hemoglobin level was 13.6 g with a standard deviation (measure of variability) of 1.2 g. For the 38 Bull Durham's patients, the mean hemoglobin level was 12.6 g with a standard deviation of 0.8. The *t* value or *t* statistic computed for these data turns out to be 4.0. Checking in the *t* table of a standard statistical text, and using the size of our samples as a guide, we find that the probability (*P* value) of obtaining a *t* value of this magnitude or greater is only .0001. In other words, given the size of our samples and the variability of the data, we would expect to see a difference between estimated means as large as the one we observe only 1 in 10,000 times if the null hypothesis were true and both samples were derived from the same population. Thus, it seems unlikely that sampling variability is responsible for our results, and we decide that in fact our Lydia Pinkham's patients have higher hemoglobin levels than those who received Bull Durham's Extract.

Another way of assessing our result is to construct one of the confidence intervals described in the previous chapter. A 95% confidence interval turns out to be 0.5–1.4. This means that our estimate for the true difference in hemoglobin levels is consistent with a range between 0.5 and 1.4 g. This interval does not contain 0 g, that is, no difference, between the groups.

CORRELATION

Correlation is another commonly encountered statistical procedure. Correlation evaluates the strength of linear relationships or associations between variables. How closely are patients' weights and blood pressures related to one another? Is the time patients spend in the waiting room linked to their satisfaction? Does the risk of acquiring AIDS increase with the number of blood transfusions a patient receives? With correlation, we observe how the changes in one variable, such as blood pressure or satisfaction, are related to changes in a second measure, such as weight or waiting time. For every incremental increase or decrease in kilograms or minutes spent in the waiting room, is there a predictable increase or decrease in millimeters of mercury of systolic blood pressure or levels of satisfaction on a self-rating questionnaire?

The concept of correlation is depicted graphically in Figure 9-2. The scatterplot of data in this figure displays a relationship between the variables "weight" on the x axis and "blood pressure" on the y axis. As x increases in value, so does y. The statistic that summarizes this relationship is called the *correlation coefficient,* symbolized by r. Several tests of correlation are commonly used, depending on the distribution of data being analyzed. The coefficient characterizes the relationship between the x and y variables. The closer values cluster in a linear relationship, the higher the correlation coefficient and the greater the association between x and y. Correlation coefficients range between -1 and $+1$. If one value decreases while another increases, the coefficient is negative. So r is commonly expressed as .56, $-.10$, and so on. The closer a correlation coefficient is to 1.0 (or to -1.0), the more strongly associated the data. As with other relationships, there are tests to determine whether correlations are "statistically significant." On the basis of the numbers of observations and the variability of the data, how likely is it that the observed association is due to chance? Correlation coefficients are usually reported together with the familiar P value. In the case of the data shown in Figure 9–2,

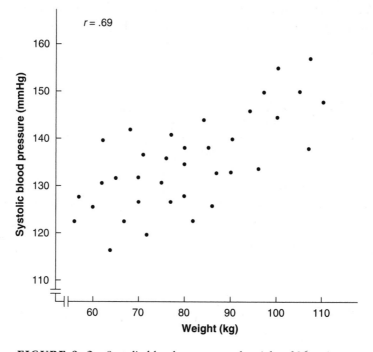

FIGURE 9–2. Systolic blood pressure and weight of 36 patients.

the correlation coefficient is .69, indicating a strong, positive relationship between weight and systolic blood pressure. The value of P is less than .001, suggesting that the association is unlikely to be due to quirks of sampling.

As another example, let us examine an observation that several medical students have made that there are differences in the way residents and faculty evaluate students on the internal medicine service. The students feel that faculty ratings are heavily influenced by the demonstration of knowledge, while residents consider other aspects of work performance as well. The students are willing to wager that if we compare clinical grades given by faculty and residents with student results on standardized knowledge-based examinations, we will see a strong relationship between performance on the knowledge-based exams and faculty ratings.

Intrigued by this hypothesis, we collect evaluation data on the last 36 students who completed the internal medicine rotation. A partial list of these data is shown in Table 9–3. It is difficult to determine much from data organized in the manner shown in the table, so we construct two scatterplots to help us visualize the relationships. The upper scatterplot in Figure 9–3 depicts the association between faculty grades (on the y axis) and examination scores (on the x axis); the lower scatterplot shows the data for resident grades and examination scores. Both plots suggest a positive

TABLE 9–3

Clinical ratings of faculty and residents compared with examination scores for 36 students (partial list)

| Student | Clinical rating | | Examination score |
	Faculty	Resident	
A	86	90	520
B	85	86	530
C	87	88	445
D	89	85	580
E	94	96	680
F	84	82	430
–	–	–	–
–	–	–	–

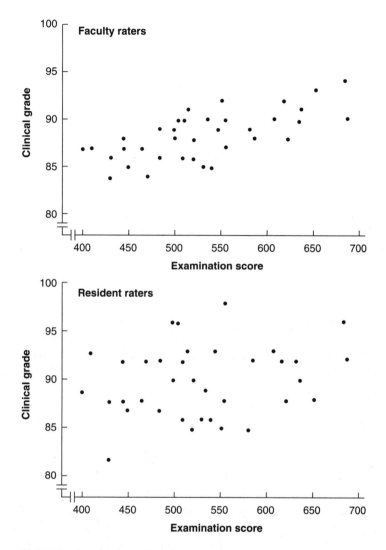

FIGURE 9–3. Clinical grades given by faculty and resident raters and examination scores for 36 medical students.

relationship that higher examination scores are associated with higher clinical grades. However, the points are more tightly clustered and thus the relationship appears to be stronger for faculty grades and exam scores.

This relationship can also be summarized statistically by calculating a correlation coefficient for each set of data. The Pearson coefficient r is .66 for the data depicting faculty grades and examination scores and .21

for the data showing resident grades and examination scores. These coefficients support the associations suggested in the scatterplots. Faculty grading appears more closely related to cognitive examination results than does resident grading. The data support (though certainly do not prove) the students' hypothesis.

REGRESSION

Correlation belongs to a larger class of statistical techniques known as regression. *Regression analysis* works on the principle we have just examined. A line is fitted to a group of data to describe relationships between variables. However, regression analysis can be put to more ambitious purposes than simply addressing the strength of the associations. Regression techniques can provide details about the association. As patients gain weight, systolic blood pressure rises. But how much? If all our patients gained 10 kg, how much would the average blood pressure rise? Or, more important, if each of our overweight patients lost 10 or 20 kg, what kind of a reduction in blood pressure might we expect? Simple correlation coefficients are unit-free; that is, they measure the strength of a relationship but do not describe the magnitude of change among variables. Regression models do this. For every kilogram that body weight changes, systolic pressure changes 0.4 mmHg, on average.

Regression techniques are also employed to create diagnostic and therapeutic predictive models. These can sort through groups of variables and consider the role of several factors simultaneously to predict clinical outcomes. Which items of history and physical exam contribute most to predicting the patients with sore throat who will have streptococcal pharyngitis? What clinical and laboratory information best identifies patients at risk for deep venous thrombosis after major abdominal surgery? What groups of symptoms and electrocardiographic findings best discriminate chest-pain patients who have myocardial ischemia from those with noncardiac pain? Regression models can evaluate several potential predictors, such as fever, tonsillar exudates, tender cervical nodes, antithrombin III concentration, substernal location of pain, and ST-segment depression, to determine which contribute significantly to identifying patients who have streptococcal pharyngitis, are at risk of deep venous thrombosis, or need admission to the coronary care unit.

They can also tell us the relative amount or weight each variable contributes to predicting the outcome of interest.

There are several variations on the regression theme. A reader will encounter intimidating terms such as "logistic regression," "discriminate function analysis," "log linear models," and "stepwise multiple regression." These are all forms of regression procedures that involve manipulating multiple variables simultaneously to determine which best predicts the outcome.

An example of this useful technique is found in a paper from the osteoporosis literature.[1] Diagnosing this asymptomatic condition is problematic. The most effective aid available is the bone densitometer. Bone mineral density (BMD) has a high correlation with the presence of osteoporosis and subsequent risk of osteoporosis-related fractures. However, the test is expensive. Investigators wondered if a simple patient questionnaire could elicit risk factors that would identify those who would most benefit from densitometry. They found over 1200 postmenopausal women from 106 physician practices. The women completed a questionnaire of approximately 60 items relating to body mass, lifestyle, reproductive history, current medical conditions, and medications. Each also had a bone density determination. On the basis of densitometry findings, subjects were categorized as having low or acceptable BMD. Potential predictive items from the questionnaire were first tested individually to see if they occurred more commonly in low BMD subjects. Items that passed were then combined in a multivariable model to see which factors best predicted the outcome when all were considered together. Only 6 items survived: race, presence of rheumatoid arthritis, history of previous fractures, older age, nonestrogen use, and low weight, as seen in Table 9–4.

The authors then assigned each factor a numeric weight based on its contribution to the model. An individual's score was calculated by summing the numeric weights for each factor present (see Table 9–4). Scores ranged from –8 to +28; the higher the number, the greater the risk of low BMD. To find the best referral strategy, researchers looked for a dividing line in the array of scores that would maximize correct referrals (send women who indeed had low BMD to get the test, but spare those with acceptable levels). When a cut point of 6 was selected, 89% of subjects with low BMD were referred while 50% with acceptable BMD levels were spared an unnecessary examination.

Regression models add more statistical nomenclature to the reader's vocabulary. Each variable that contributes to the predictive model will have its own *coefficient*. This may be a positive or negative number and

	TABLE 9–4	
	Coefficients for calculating SCORE **(Simple Calculated Osteoporosis Risk Estimation)**	
Variable	**Score**	**If woman**
Race	5	is NOT Black
Rheumatoid arthritis	4	HAS rheumatoid arthritis
History of fractures	4	For EACH TYPE (wrist, rib, hip) of nontraumatic fracture after age 45 (maximum score = 12)
Age	3	× first digit of age in years
Estrogen	1	if NEVER received estrogen therapy
Weight	−1	× weight ÷ by 10 and truncated to integer

SCORE equals sum of above.
Example: A 126-lb, 67-year-old White woman with a history of rheumatoid arthritis, no history of fractures, and a history of estrogen therapy would have a SCORE of 15, or 5 (for race) + 4 (for rheumatoid arthritis) + (4 × 0) (for no history of fracture) + (3 × 6) (for age) + 0 (for previous estrogen therapy) − (1 × 12) (for weight). Since 15 is greater than the threshold score of 6, this woman should be referred for bone densitometry.
Modified, with permission, from Lydick et al.[1]

simply indicates the weighting the variable has in the model. For the scatterplot depicting the relationship between weight and systolic blood pressure, the regression equation BP = 99 + .45 (weight in kilograms) describes the relationship mathematically (Figure 9–4). The general form of this equation is $y = a + bx$, where a is the theoretical point of intercept on the y axis when x is equal to zero, and b is the amount of change in the y variable for every unit change of x. Practically speaking, this means that we can predict, on average, our patients' systolic blood pressures from their weights. Starting with 99-mmHg of pressure, we add 0.45 times weight to derive systolic pressure. In other words, for every additional kilogram of weight, blood pressure increases almost 0.5 mm. Remember, of course, that the equation is simply our best summary estimate of the blood pressure–weight relationship and that individual patient values will vary from the model just as they do in the scatterplot.

A term that is often used in describing correlation and regression relationships is r^2—the square of the correlation coefficient r. It is interpreted as representing the amount of variance in an outcome variable (such as blood pressure) that can be attributed to changes in a predictor

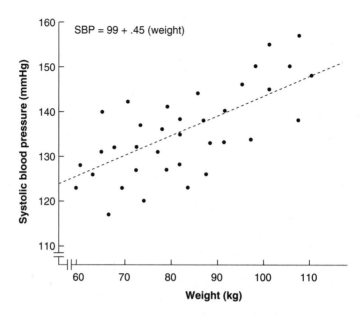

FIGURE 9–4. Systolic blood pressure (SBP) and weight of 36 patients.

variable (such as weight). In our example, the correlation coefficient r was .69. Squaring r, we obtain a value of .48, which we can interpret as indicating that 48% of the variance in the patient's blood pressure is related to weight. Stated another way, differences in weight predict almost half of the variability we observe in blood pressures. The remaining 52% is due to other factors.

This means that correlation coefficients must be relatively high (close to 1.0) before the association they describe can be said to predict or explain a substantial proportion of the outcome. If we were to find, for example, that length of waiting time in the doctor's office correlates with patient satisfaction with $r = .3$, our results would indicate that only 9% ($.3^2$) of patient satisfaction has been explained by length of wait.

SUMMARY

Understanding the principles that guide the selection and application of statistical tests aids critical reading. When researchers use appropriate tests to analyze their ordinal data or successfully use regression models to sort through a confusing array of predictor variables to help us decide when bone density examinations are indicated, their results gain credibility. Several tips are worth remembering:

1. Many medical researchers now consider the services of a biostatistician essential in helping with the design and analysis of the study. It is worth browsing through the roster of authors to identify PhD degrees that may indicate advanced statistical training and perusing the list of author affiliations to see if departments of statistics have been involved. Sometimes statistical assistance is indicated only by an acknowledgment at the end of the paper.

2. The principles of sound study design still apply. No statistical tests can transform poor data into useful information. If subjects are unwittingly selected because they are sicker or healthier or more cooperative, if blood pressures are measured by a biased observer, or if there are differing levels of regimen compliance because Lydia Pinkham's Compound tastes better than Bull Durham's Extract, the most sophisticated regression model will not help.

3. Several general-readership journals publish feature articles that review statistical topics. These are worth reading and saving as aids to critical review.

4. Statistical significance still does not mean clinical importance.

REFERENCE

1. Lydick E et al: Development and validation of a simple questionnaire to facilitate identification of women likely to have low bone density. Am J Manag Care 1998;4(1):37.

CHAPTER TEN

Interpretation: Sensitivity, Specificity, and Predictive Value

You pays your money and you takes your choice.

PUNCH

We live with a surfeit of choices. The mail brings almost daily suggestions for enriching our medical knowledge while we are cruising through Caribbean islands or skiing in the Wasatch Mountains. Journals offer multicolored proposals from pharmaceutical companies for reducing patient blood pressures or relieving contact dermatitis—mixed in with the latest epidemiologic pronouncements on the causes of cancer. Suggestions for improving our diagnostic capabilities are also abundant. Descriptive studies and cross-sectional designs touting clinical signs and symptoms, laboratory determinations, and radiographic procedures as aids in clinical decision making are much in vogue. Magnetic resonance imaging and ultrasound devices claim to localize lacunae in our heads, holes in our hearts, and cysts in our kidneys. Old techniques such as the C-reactive protein are revitalized and used to diagnose vascular inflammation. Clinical signs and symptoms are combined in different ways in an effort to best predict when stool cultures are likely to yield enteric

177

pathogens. With all the new and not-so-new technological approaches available, it is difficult to decide which dishes among the diagnostic smorgasbord are most worthwhile. In this chapter, we will devote ourselves to interpreting evaluations of these diagnostic ideas and prediction tools.

There are several approaches to assigning value to a new test or clinical complex. The first, which is encountered with distressing frequency, is the author's proclamation that it is so. "In my experience, right upper quadrant pain means cholecystitis." "We have found that bilateral infiltrates on chest radiographs signify Legionnaire's disease." The presence of gallbladder disease in 8 out of 10 patients with abdominal pain, or the observation that the last 5 patients with chest films that had patchy infiltrates had antibody titers to *Legionella*, are "swallows that do not a summer make." Uncontrolled observations filter into the most respected of publications. They may be useful as preliminary, descriptive hunches but should be challenged to provide evidence of validity and generalizability. "Author" and "authority" come from common Middle English stock and run the danger of becoming synonyms in the minds of some.

A somewhat more satisfactory approach to assessing a new diagnostic technique is to employ a statistical test of association to see if the new method helps discover disease more often than might be expected by chance. The article on blood culturing and bacteremia relies on P values and statistical significance to support its claims for diagnostic effectiveness.[1] Recall that one of the tidbits of information imparted from this study was that certain clinical and laboratory features were useful predictors of which children would ultimately be found to have bacteremia. Among these were age, fever, and white blood cell (WBC) count (see Table 10–1).

> Bacteremia was most frequent in children 7–12 months old ($P < 0.001$) and was associated with a white cell count of 20,000 or more ($P < 0.01$) and a temperature of 39.4°C or higher ($P < 0.01$).[1]

Shunning the seduction of the small P value and remembering that statistically significant predictors may not be clinically useful guides, we find that Table 10–1 provides some helpful information. The frequency of positive blood cultures does rise with temperature as well as with WBC count and is higher in one of the younger age groups. It also appears that this observation is unlikely to be due to chance. But somehow we are not getting the complete picture. We know something of how valuable the temperature and WBC count are in predicting disease when they are elevated: About 12% of the time, a high WBC count will identify a patient

TABLE 10–1			
Factors associated with bacteremia in febrile pediatric outpatients			
Factor	Positive cultures	Total cultures	Percent positive
Age (months)			
6 or younger	1	74	1.4
7–12	11	116	9.5
13–24	5	131	3.8
25 or older	5	225	2.2
Temperature (°C)			
<38.9	2	159	1.3
38.9–39.4	4	99	4.0
39.4–39.9 (sic)	10	124	8.1
40.0 or higher	6	96	6.3
White blood cell count			
($\times 10^3$/mm^3)			
<10.0	2	162	1.2
10.0–19.9	13	193	6.7
20.0 or more	6	52	11.5

Modified, with permission, from McGowan et al.[1]

with bacteremia; 7% of the time, a temperature of 39.4°C or higher will accurately predict the problem. It is also clear, however, that these tests are not always right; they are correct only 12 and 7% of the time. That means that 88 of 100 and 93 of 100 times, a high WBC count and a high fever incorrectly suggest that patients have bacteremia. Furthermore, the tests also fail to detect some patients who have disease. Not every patient who is bacteremic meets the criterion of temperature higher than 39.4°C or WBC count above 20,000/mm^3. These are important errors in classification and are limitations in the tests that clinicians must incorporate into decision making. Pronouncements of statistical significance alone do not provide sufficient information.

Recasting some of the data contained in Table 10–1 into the schematic seen in Table 10–2 provides us with a better sense of how the tests are performing. A temperature of 39.4°C or higher occurs in 220 of 478 patients. Sixteen of these children turn out to have bacteremia, for a frequency of about 7%. However, we can see from the table that 6 children who have positive blood cultures have temperatures below 39.4°C.

TABLE 10−2							
Factors associated with bacteremia in febrile pediatric outpatients							
Temperature, °C (temp)				**White blood cells/mm³ (WBC)**			
	Blood culture				Blood culture		
	Positive	Negative	Total		Positive	Negative	Total
Temp ≥39.4°C	16	204	220	WBC ≥20,000	6	46	52
<39.4°C	6	252	258	<20,000	15	340	355
	22	456	478		21	386	407

Modified, with permission, from McGowan et al.[1]

These children will be misclassified by the criterion of high fever. It is also apparent from inspecting the tables that while 252 of the 456 children who did not have bacteremia are correctly classified by the criterion of temperature below 39.4°C, a substantial number, 204, are incorrectly labeled as bacteremic. Similarly, a WBC count above 20,000/mm³ is an accurate predictor of bacteremia on 6 of 52 occasions, or 12% of the time. This test is much more accurate in identifying truly negative patients. In all, 340 of 386 children with negative blood cultures are appropriately classified by virtue of their low WBC counts. Only 46 children with negative blood cultures fall into the high WBC group and are incorrectly called bacteremic. This is a much better batting average than the temperature criterion offered. Unfortunately, the WBC count misses more cases of bacteremia than it identifies. Only 6 of 21 positive cultures have concurrent WBC counts above 20,000/mm³; 15 bacteremia patients have WBC counts that fall below the cutoff point.

We have just described a systematic approach to evaluating diagnostic tests. Concepts known as *sensitivity, specificity,* and *predictive value* are used to summarize the system. As with other bits of jargon, a moderate amount of confusion has surrounded the application of these terms. Twenty house officers, 20 fourth-year medical students, and 20 attending physicians at 4 teaching hospitals were asked in "hallway encounters" to solve a medical problem that required calculating the predictive value of a test.[2] Only 11 of the 60 participants were able to come up with the correct answer. The reasoning is straightforward in the sensitivity, specificity, and predictive-value game, but it takes a bit of thought to digest the principles and—for most of us—a pencil and piece of paper for sketching a hasty two-by-two table like the one shown in Table 10–3.

Sensitivity is the ability of a test to single out people who have disease. For those who thrive on equations, using the notations in Table 10–3, sensitivity is $A/(A + C)$. *Specificity* is the ability of the test to classify people who do not have illness as negative. In the algebra of Table 10–3, it is $D/(B + D)$. The *predictive value* of a diagnostic endeavor gives the frequency with which a positive test actually signifies disease. Reading horizontally across Table 10–3, it is $A/(A + B)$. Predictive value is more properly designated as *positive predictive value* (the value of a positive test). Its companion, *negative predictive value*—the frequency with which a negative test identifies people without disease—is substantially less useful. Most authors are speaking positively when they refer to predictive value.

Let us return to the bacteremia data and attach some terms to the information we compiled. Table 10–4 summarizes the sensitivity, specificity, and predictive value for temperature and WBC count as diagnostic tests for bacteremia. The 2 tests may be compared, and the intuitive reservations we developed from examining Table 10–2 can be quantified. Using temperature to diagnose bacteremia, we will properly identify 73% of patients who have positive cultures. That is the sensitivity. Our specificity is not very high; only 55% of patients who are without disease will be properly identified by their position in the lower-temperature group.

TABLE 10–3
Sensitivity, specificity, and predictive value

		Disease		
		Present	Absent	
Test	Positive	A	B	$A + B$
	Negative	C	D	$C + D$
		$A + C$	$B + D$	$A + B + C + D$
	Sensitivity	$= A/(A + C)$		
	Specificity	$= D/(B + D)$		
	Predictive value	$= A/(A + B)$		

TABLE 10-4

Sensitivity, specificity, and predictive value of temperature and WBC count in diagnosing bacteremia

Temperature, °C (temp)				White blood cells/mm³ (WBC)			
	Blood culture				Blood culture		
	Positive	Negative	Total		Positive	Negative	Total
Temp ≥39.4°C	16	204	220	WBC ≥20,000	6	46	52
<39.4°C	6	252	258	<20,000	15	340	355
	22	456	478		21	386	407

Sensitivity	= 16/22 = 73%	Sensitivity	= 6/21 = 29%
Specificity	= 252/456 = 55%	Specificity	= 340/386 = 88%
Predictive value	= 16/220 = 7%	Predictive value	= 6/52 = 12%

Modified, with permission, from McGowan et al.[1]

The predictive value of fever is low; only 7% of all children with temperatures above 39.4°C will have positive blood cultures. The specificity of the WBC count, 88%, is much better. Sensitivity, however, suffers when this test is used; only 29% of children with positive cultures are properly identified. The WBC count offers better predictive value: Of the 52 children with elevated WBC counts, 12% have bacteremia.

There is a message in all this. Diagnostic tests are not perfect. Some degree of misclassification of patients is inevitable. By using attributes of sensitivity, specificity, and predictive value, we are able to quantify in a standard way the ability of any test to make correct and incorrect classifications. Some papers will speak of the efficiency of a test. *Efficiency* is an overall estimate of a test's ability to classify patients correctly. The boxes in Table 10–4 surround the numbers of patients who are correctly labeled. Efficiency is the combination of these 2 correct classification boxes divided by the total number of patients assessed. For temperature, this would be (16 + 252)/478, or 56%; for WBC count, the efficiency is (6 + 340)/407, or 85%.

The concept of efficiency may overly summarize the attributes of the test. White blood cell count appears to be a more efficient diagnostic test than temperature for detecting bacteremia. But how concerned is the clinician about missing cases of bacteremia? The high efficiency of WBC count is due largely to the fact that most patients have negative cultures and also have WBC counts below 20,000/mm^3. Over two-thirds of positive cultures are misidentified by using the criterion of the elevated WBC count. Sensitivity this low is not acceptable. If a disease is worth detecting, a 71% miss, or *false-negative,* rate is unacceptable. Elevated temperature is a more sensitive test; only about one-fourth of patients with positive cultures will fall into the false-negative category. On the other hand, when we choose fever, specificity suffers. Elevated temperatures were seen in 204 of the 456 patients with negative cultures. These are *false positives*, test results falsely indicating the presence of disease.

PREVALENCE

The purpose of a diagnostic test is to improve our level of certainty about the cause of a patient's illness. Sensitivity and specificity are useful gauges of a test's value. The higher these numbers, the better the test. However, there are other factors to consider. The frequency, or *prevalence,* of the condition or disease in the population being tested is a major concern. Readers will encounter references to the pretest, or prior, probability and to posttest, or posterior, probability in discussions of diagnostic procedures. *Pretest,* or *prior, probability* is the prevalence of a condition in the study population. A pretest probability of 5% means that 5 of every 100 subjects in the total group being tested will have the condition. Thus our chances of correctly guessing the diagnosis *without* the benefit of diagnostic devices is 5%. *Posttest,* or *posterior, probability* is the same as predictive value. We hope that after we know a test is positive, our ability to predict the presence of disease in that subgroup will be enhanced. Conversely, a negative test should result in a marked decrease in likelihood of disease from the pretest probability.

Table 10–5 shows the benefit of a positive diagnostic test that has a 90% sensitivity and 90% specificity for a disease with a pretest probability of 5%. The bottom row of the table indicates that 100 of every 2000 subjects tested (5%) have the disease in question (prevalence/pretest probability). Of those 2000 individuals, 280 will have a positive test (top row), and 90 of those who test positive will actually have disease. The ratio of 90/280 (32%) is the predictive value/posttest probability of a positive test and

TABLE 10-5
Prevalence/pretest probability and predictive value/posttest probability

		Disease		
		Present	Absent	
Test	Positive	90	190	280
	Negative	10	1710	1720
		100	1900	2000

Sensitivity	= 90/100	= 90%
Specificity	= 1710/1900	= 90%
Prevalence	= 100/2000	= 5%
Predictive value	= 90/280	= 32%

represents a sixfold improvement over the pretest level. The high sensitivity and specificity have worked to produce a test that enhances diagnosis.

However, in some situations, where pretest probability/prevalence is very low, the value of tests with even high sensitivity and specificity may be reduced. Policies proposed by state legislatures to require mandatory premarital serologic testing for HIV prompted researchers from Boston to estimate the benefits of a premarital screening program.[3] Initial screening was to be done with an enzyme immunoassay (EIA) that the authors estimated had a sensitivity of 98.3% and a specificity of 99.8%. These are impressive numbers indeed. It is hard to find a more accurate test in any arsenal. The key to the analysis, however, is the estimate of the prevalence or pretest probability of HIV. As we saw in Chapter 4, these prevalence estimates vary widely. Since no data were available on the actual frequency of HIV among the premarital population, the authors used information derived from blood donors. The figure they came up with was only 35 positives for every 100,000 individuals tested. When test characteristics and this pretest probability are applied to the almost 4 million individuals who are married each year, the expected distribution of results is as seen in Table 10–6.

Despite the high levels of sensitivity and specificity, the very low prevalence of HIV infection in the premarital population creates a posttest probability of only 15%. This means that for every 1300 individuals

TABLE 10-6 Expected enzyme immunoassay results in 1-year premarital screening program			
	HIV infection	**No infection**	**HIV total**
Positive	1325	7648	8973
Negative	23	3,816,372	3,816,395
Total	1348	3,824,020	3,825,368

Sensitivity	= 1325/1348	= 98.3%
Specificity	= 3,816,372/3,824,020	= 99.8%
Prevalence	= 1348/3,825,368	= .035%
Predictive value	= 1325/8973	= 14.8%

Modified, with permission, from Cleary et al.[3]

correctly diagnosed as HIV-infected, there are over 7600 false positives. That is a great many people who will be unnecessarily alarmed by the specter of HIV.

The authors employed a second stage to the screening and submitted EIA-positive individuals to a confirming test, the Western blot. The Western blot also has excellent test characteristics, with a sensitivity of 92% and specificity of 95%. But even after this second round, over 380 people remained falsely classified as HIV-positive. There is an important message here. Prevalence, or pretest probability, is critical to any screening or case-finding exercise. One needs to identify subjects with as high a pretest probability as possible before testing begins. In the case of HIV testing, subjects in a general premarital population who lack identified risk factors for HIV infection are not reasonable candidates for screening.*

---

*Despite the concerns raised by the Boston study,[3] Illinois instituted premarital HIV testing. Results of the first 6 months of the program were reported, and the yield of positive tests was even less than estimated.[4] Only 8 of more than 70,000 marriage-license applicants were seropositive, for a frequency of 11 per 100,000. The estimated cost of the program was $2.5 million, or about $312,000 for every positive applicant.

MAKING CHOICES

The game of diagnostics is one of trade-offs. When we attempt to improve the sensitivity of our procedures and detect everyone who has an illness, we become less selective. We fall back on the most common denominator, like fever, and include people who do not have the disease. We can become more restrictive by raising the specificity of the test and reducing the number of false-positive determinations. But then sensitivity is bound to suffer.

Nevertheless, choices between sensitivity and specificity must be made. How do we decide where to draw the line between positive and negative and between sensitivity and specificity? The answer is not a statistical one. It is a clinical and economic decision. What are the costs of misclassifying patients? When the consequences of missing a disease are crucial, as in the case of a curable cancer or treatable, life-threatening bacterial infection, sensitivity is paramount. We are willing to risk misclassifying a few people as positives, especially if other, more definitive diagnostic procedures are available to correct our initial mistakes.

Screening programs to detect phenylketonuria (PKU) among newborns attempt to be very sensitive. Failure to detect cases of this treatable genetic disease will result in permanent mental retardation and great personal and social cost. A percentage of false positives will occur in these screening programs, but repeated blood tests are readily available to reclassify these babies correctly.

If, on the other hand, the burden of creating false positives outweighs the advantages of capturing all cases of a disease, increasing specificity should be the goal. If exploratory surgery or invasive angiography is necessary to confirm a diagnosis, high specificity is desirable. An example of a clinical sign that is frequently encountered and should be specific is the heart murmur. While the heart murmur can be a reasonably sensitive diagnostic aid for detecting valvular heart disease (most people with bad valves have murmurs), there are many people who have murmurs and perfectly normal hearts (false positives). Substantial medical costs can be incurred if extensive cardiac evaluation is performed on every patient who has a murmur. Thousands of cardiograms, ultrasound examinations, and even catheterizations can be done to document the absence of heart disease in patients misclassified by the presence of a murmur. Bergman and Stamm have even written about the psychological effects that can occur when children with "innocent" heart murmurs are thought by parents to have heart disease.[5] Activities become restricted as children are put into undesirable sick roles by diagnostic misclassification.

When tests are repeated over time, false positives may accumulate. Elmore et al used a retrospective cohort approach to follow up on 2400 women who were enrollees in a large health maintenance organization that promoted breast cancer screening.[6] Women over the age of 40 were encouraged to have mammograms and clinical breast examinations on a regular basis. The 2400 women were followed up for 10 years, during which time 9762 screening mammograms were performed. The median number of mammograms per subject over the interval was 4. False-positive reports were considered those that created a suspicion of cancer but where the diagnosis was not confirmed after further follow-up.

Overall, the mammograms had good specificity, about 93.5%. That means that only 6.5% of those without breast cancer are labeled as false positive. But when women have repeated tests, as they do in the screening programs, the likelihood of any individual encountering a false-positive result increases. Overall, almost 24% of women who participated in the mammography screening had at least one false-positive test. The likelihood of a false positive increases with the number of mammograms the subject has. Among the small number of women in the study who had as many as 9 mammograms, over 40% encountered at least 1 false positive. Such misclassifications bring with them considerable anxiety and added medical costs. Additional workups following the false-positive mammograms included outpatient visits, diagnostic imaging, and biopsies. The authors report that for every $100 spent on the screening program, an added $33 of expense was incurred to evaluate the false-positive results.

LIKELIHOOD RATIOS

Although this chapter seems to contain a surfeit of new terminology, there is more to come. Further assistance in describing and making choices among tests is offered by the *likelihood ratio* (*LR*). The likelihood ratio addresses the question, "How much more likely are we to find that a test is positive among patients with disease compared with those without disease?" It is an indication of the test's discriminatory power and is constructed as a ratio of the proportion of patients with disease who test positive to those who test positive but are without disease. (Technically speaking, this is the likelihood ratio of a positive as opposed to a negative test.) Invoking the terminology we have just learned, this likelihood ratio positive is the ratio of sensitivity to 1 − specificity. When a test has high sensitivity as well as high specificity (1 − specificity is low), the likelihood ratio is high and discrimination is good. An obvious advantage of the likelihood ratio is its ability to summarize the relationship between sensitivity and specificity in a single number. This gives readers an easy way to compare the discriminatory capabilities of tests.

Likelihood ratios have been used to sort the relative merits of the signs and symptoms used to identify patients with appendicitis. Many clinicians have learned a rather lengthy list of clinical clues that help decide whether a patient with abdominal pain has an inflamed appendix. Most lists feature such findings as right lower quadrant pain, rebound tenderness, fever, vomiting, rectal tenderness, and migratory pain for starters. But often no distinction is made as to which of these is most important, which best sorts those with appendicitis from those without the condition. Wagner et al performed an extensive literature review to determine the predictive abilities of signs and symptoms to identify appendicitis.[7] A list, based on their determinations, is seen in Table 10–7. The table shows the sensitivity and specificity of each finding as well as quite a range of positive likelihood ratios. Right lower quadrant pain,

---

TABLE 10–7

Sensitivity, specificity, and likelihood ratio + (LR+) of clinical examination findings for appendicitis[a]

Finding	Sensitivity	Specificity	LR+
Right lower quadrant pain	0.84	0.89	7.6
Internal rigidity	0.32	0.91	3.6
Migration	0.75	0.79	3.6
Fever	0.67	0.79	3.2
Rebound tenderness	0.63	0.69	2.0
Guarding	0.74	0.57	1.7
Nausea	0.58	0.37	0.9
Vomiting	0.51	0.45	0.9

[a]Data have been modified for instructional purposes.
Modified, with permission, from Wagner et al.[7]

rigidity, and the migration of pain from the periumbilical region to the right lower quadrant show good discrimination. Symptoms of nausea and vomiting are not particularly helpful.

However, while there is benefit to the summarizing property of likelihood ratios (one number to think about instead of two), there is also a liability. A test's discriminating ability does not tell the whole story. Look at migration of pain and abdominal rigidity in the table. Both have reasonable discriminating power; they are 3.6 times more likely to be found in patients with appendicitis than in those without. But while the ratios are similar, sensitivities are not. Migration occurs among 75% of patients with appendicitis while rigidity is present in only 32% of cases. Because rigidity has particularly good specificity (91%) and its occurrence in subjects without appendicitis is low, the likelihood ratio is reasonable (0.32 ÷ 0.09 = 3.6). Migration shows similar discriminating ability (likelihood ratio) because, although sensitivity is higher (75%), specificity is only 79% (so, 1 − specificity = 21). The 2 signs are equally helpful in distinguishing appendicitis from nonappendicitis when they are *present* but not when *absent*. This is because of the poor sensitivity of rigidity (high false negatives). A test that is only positive in 32% of cases is of limited value no matter how good its positive likelihood ratio may be.

Working with tests where results are dichotomous, that is, either present or absent, positive or negative, is reasonably straightforward. There are many situations, however, in which we are confronted with a range of values—hemoglobin levels to define anemia or a prostate-specific antigen value that suggests prostate cancer—where decisions become more complex. We must decide not only which tests to use but also which values of a test best serve our purposes. Let us return to the example of the 6-item questionnaire that was developed to predict low bone mineral density (BMD).[8]

Recall that Lydick et al developed this self-administered, 6-item survey to identify patients at high risk of osteoporosis who should be referred for BMD examination. Each item in the scale was given a weight and each patient a composite score based on her responses. In developing the Simple Calculated Osteoporosis Risk Estimation (SCORE) instrument, the investigators compared questionnaire results with measured BMD in 1246 patients. SCORE scores ranged from −4 to +20, with highest scores indicating a greater likelihood of low BMD and osteoporosis. The question becomes "Where in this array of SCORE values does one 'draw the line' and decide a referral is necessary?" Table 10–8 offers data on sensitivity, specificity, and positive likelihood ratio for possible

TABLE 10-8

**Sensitivity, specificity, 1 - specificity, and likelihood ratio + (LR +)
for selected SCORE thresholds**

	Sensitivity	Specificity	1 - Specificity	LR+
0	0.99	0.12	0.88	1.1
1	0.99	0.17	0.83	1.2
2	0.98	0.20	0.80	1.2
3	0.97	0.26	0.74	1.3
4	0.94	0.34	0.66	1.4
5	0.93	0.42	0.58	1.6
6	0.89	0.50	0.50	1.8
7	0.82	0.58	0.42	1.9
8	0.74	0.67	0.33	2.2
9	0.67	0.75	0.25	2.7
10	0.60	0.82	0.18	3.4

SCORE, Simple Calculated Osteoporosis Risk Estimation.
Modified, with permission, from Lydick et al.[8]

SCORE thresholds from 0 to 10. If a threshold of 4 were used, for example, all patients with scores of 4 or higher would be referred.

The table confronts us with trade-offs. Lower values for SCORE (5 or less) have high sensitivity, 90% or better, but sacrifice specificity, with values of 40% or less. This means many false positives will be referred. Likelihood ratios are also low, indicating little discrimination. We can, of course, move the threshold to favor higher specificity and fewer false positives. Sensitivity then suffers. How is one to choose?

Let us look at 3 possible threshold options in tabular form to see if more detail is enlightening (see Table 10-9). We see that there are some advantages to each of the thresholds shown. A threshold of 3 or more has a very high sensitivity (97%); only 16 of 473 women with low BMD are not referred. The downside is low specificity (only 26%). A high false-positive rate results in 75% of individuals who have adequate BMD being referred. With the high number of false positives, positive predictive value suffers as well. The prevalence, or prior probability, in this group of subjects is .38 (473/1246). The threshold of 3 classifies 1031 as needing referral, but only 44% (457) of those actually have low BMD (predictive value positive).

TABLE 10-9					
Three possible SCORE thresholds for determining referral for bone mineral density (BMD) examination					
	SCORE threshold 3+ BMD		SCORE threshold 6+ BMD		SCORE threshold 9+ BMD
SCORE	Low	Acceptable	Low	Acceptable	Low	Acceptable
Threshold or higher	457	574	423	389	319	196
Below threshold	16	199	50	384	154	577
	473	773	473	773	473	773
Sensitivity	457/473 = .97		423/473 = .89		319/473 = .67	
Specificity	199/773 = .26		384/773 = .50		577/773 = .75	
Likelihood ratio +	.97/.74 = 1.2		.89/.50 = 1.8		.67/.25 = 2.7	
Predictive value +	457/1031 = .44		423/812 = .52		319/515 = .62	
Prevalence (prior probability)			473/1246 = .38			

SCORE, Simple Calculated Osteoporosis Risk Estimation.
Modified, with permission, from Lydick et al.[8]

Moving to a threshold of 9 improves specificity considerably (75%) and reduces false positives to only 196. This lower number helps raise the positive likelihood ratio (2.7) and the positive predictive value (.62). The problem is that sensitivity falls to 67%, meaning that one-third of women needing referral will not get it. That is not acceptable to the investigators. They make the decision to require a minimum sensitivity of about 90% and choose a threshold of 6, meaning that they are unwilling to miss (fail to refer) more than 10% of subjects who have low BMD. That means they take some lumps on specificity—only 50%. Still, they have a likelihood ratio of 1.8 and a positive predictive value of .52, some evidence of discrimination, and an improvement over the prior probability of .38. As the investigators' initial goal was to develop an instrument that would improve referrals for BMD examination, SCORE with a threshold of 6 is a moderate success. Of the 1200 subjects evaluated, almost 90% of the 473 with low BMD were appropriately referred, while 384 were spared unnecessary referral.

ROC CURVES

Still another way of depicting data is by the *receiver operator character-istic (ROC)* curve, a concept borrowed from psychologists and engineers. An ROC curve portraying the SCORE data is seen in Figure 10–1. The curve illustrates the trade-offs as sensitivity (displayed on the *y* axis) increases; 1 – specificity (the false positives) also rises. The threshold points we have discussed are indicated on the curve. In general, the best threshold choices reside on the upper left-hand side, where sensitivity is high but 1 – specificity is low. As one moves down and to the left from this point, sensitivity falls disproportionate to the gains in specificity. By the same token, as one moves to the right, the curve flattens out and, for a very minor gain in sensitivity, much specificity is lost (1 – specificity rises). The diagonal line displayed on the figure connects points where sensitivity and 1 – specificity are the same; this is a line of no discrimination. As an ROC curve extends upward away from this diagonal, the test is demonstrating increasing discrimination. It is possible to calculate the

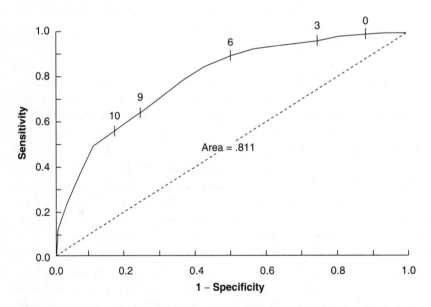

FIGURE 10–1. Receiver operator characteristic (ROC) curve for SCORE threshold values. SCORE, Simple Calculated Osteoporosis Risk Estimation. (Modified, with permission, from Lydick et al.[8])

area under this ROC curve to estimate the test's discriminatory ability. Generally speaking, when the area under the ROC curve is .8 or greater, the test provides useful discrimination.

MODELING

Lydick et al employed multivariable regression modeling to develop their SCORE instrument.[8] Many studies now use this kind of statistical approach to assist in diagnostic and therapeutic decision making and for estimating patient prognosis. Modeling can help differentiate between bacterial and viral meningitis, guide treatment decisions for patients with pharyngitis, or predict the probability of mortality for patients admitted to intensive care units. In developing their mortality prediction model for such patients, Lemeshow et al collected an array of information on 755 patients admitted to a combined medical/surgical intensive care unit.[9] Included were data on age, hospital service, blood pressure and pulse, presence of coma, infection, and cancer as well as a host of prior health conditions. The vital status of each patient at hospital discharge was also obtained. Each variable was assessed individually as a potential indicator of mortality. Those that were statistically significantly related to death or survival by a simple chi-square test became candidates for a multivariable logistic regression model. With many of the clinical variables—such as blood pressure and pulse rate—being interrelated, the statistical process helps to sort out the independent contribution of each factor and reduce the number of variables that are simply "along for the ride." Ultimately, only 7 of the 137 variables tested contributed to outcome prediction and were included in the model.

Models of this sort are useful. They help us marshal the multiple pieces of data we collect on subjects and combine them into a rational diagnostic or prognostic aid. But models have their limitations. Principles of population and sample selection still apply. When Poses et al evaluated several prediction models for streptococcal pharyngitis, they explored how well the models could be "transported" from one clinical setting to another.[10] These decision aids were developed on data obtained from patients at a student health service and combined information on fever, pharyngeal exudate, cough, and cervical node tenderness to predict the presence of strep among patients with sore throats. In their original settings, the models performed well. However, the developmental data set came from a population where the prevalence of strep infection was 15–17%. Would the models perform as well in patient groups where the rate of streptococcal infection was lower? When the tests were applied to a new group of 310 subjects in whom the culture-proven prevalence of *Streptococcus* was only 5%, the models overestimated the frequency of streptococcal infection by as much as 93%.

The investigators postulated two possible explanations for this difficulty. Either the models had lost their discriminating power in the new patient population, or the change in disease prevalence had altered the models' effectiveness. To examine the former possibility, the investigators compared ROC curve areas for the old and new study populations and found that the models performed their discriminating tasks well in both groups. This suggests that the change in prevalence had thrown predictions off kilter. Indeed, when the investigators adjusted their data statistically to match strep prevalence in the 2 populations, the models regained their predictive abilities.

The SCORE model also encountered difficulties when the recipe was taken to another venue. Investigators who were studying a population of older subjects in a community in southern California administered the instrument to over 1000 postmenopausal White women.[11] They also obtained BMD determinations on subjects. When the threshold of 6, as suggested by Lydick et al,[8] was used on this group, results were less than satisfactory. Table 10–10 displays the findings. The sensitivity is excellent, 98%, but specificity is nothing short of appalling at 13%. This means that almost 90% of subjects with acceptable BMDs fell above the threshold and were recommended for referral. In fact, of the 1013 subjects, only 5.5% escaped referral, and of those 56 individuals, 14 had low BMDs and should have been sent. The positive predictive value .69 looked rather promising until one realizes that the prevalence in this population was almost as high as .67.

In an effort to improve the SCORE's performance, investigators moved the threshold up to 11 (see Table 10–10). This maneuver has the expected result of raising specificity—up to 45%. However, we still have 55% of patients with acceptable BMDs classified as having low BMDs, and sensitivity drops to 80%. Now about 29% of subjects will not be referred for BMD testing, but unfortunately, almost half of these will have low BMDs. The test simply does not perform well in this population. Comparing the southern California group with the population on which Lydick et al developed the model uncovers some differences in risk profiles.

	TABLE 10−10			
	Application of SCORE to Rancho Bernardo cohort			
	SCORE threshold 6+ BMD		**SCORE threshold 11+ BMD**	
SCORE	Low	Acceptable	Low	Acceptable
Threshold or higher	655	292	543	184
Below threshold	14	42	136	150
	679	334	679	334
Sensitivity	665/679 = .98		543/679 = .80	
Specificity	42/334 = .13		150/334 = .45	
Likelihood ratio +	.98/.87 = 1.1		.80/.55 = 1.5	
Predictive value +	655/957 = .69		543/727 = .75	
Prevalence (prior probability)	679/1013 = .67			

SCORE, Simple Calculated Osteoporosis Risk Estimation.
Modified, with permission, from Von Muhlen et al.[11]

The southern California group, which on an average was over 10 years older, was entirely Caucasian, and had a lower frequency of estrogen use. They also had almost twice the prevalence of low BMD. Unfortunately, even when the southern California investigators repeated their analyses taking some of these population differences into account, they could still not get the SCORE model to differentiate between women with low and acceptable levels of BMD.

Caveat emptor! Even the most elegantly constructed, statistically sophisticated models travel from setting to setting at some peril.

SPECTRUM

Variations in the prevalence of a disease or makeup of the population tested influence the utility of a test, but sensitivity and specificity may also vary, depending on the clinical stage of the disease. A test that appears useful in an advanced state of illness may be less useful early in the course of the disease. This is the problem of *spectrum*.[12] Diseases are dynamic and heterogeneous in nature and present a range of manifestations and bodily reactions as they progress. The interactions between host and disease differ in early stages of illness—colon cancer, rheumatoid arthritis, or bacterial endocarditis, for example—from those that occur later on. Tests that reflect the physiology or immune response of patients with overt, symptomatic illness may have little value in preclinical cases.

Documentation of the problem of spectrum and diagnostic test utility comes from the literature on screening tests for prostate cancer. The authors of one study evaluated a radioimmunoassay for prostatic acid phosphatase in hopes that it would detect the disease early in its course, when treatment would be more effective.[13] Unfortunately, they found that the value of the test varied with the stage of progression of the cancer. In later stages of the disease, the test had reasonably high sensitivity. It identified between 71 and 92% of cancer patients. However, in the earlier stage I, only one-third of patients with known prostate cancer tested positive.

Screening for colorectal cancer with a carcinoembryonic antigen (CEA) offers another example.[14] This test is reasonably sensitive in finding advanced colorectal cancer of Duke's stages C or D, at rates of 74 and 83%, respectively. However, detection at earlier stages, where treatment is likely to be more effective, is much less successful, with a sensitivity of only 36%.

Spectrum effect has been demonstrated more broadly by a group from the Netherlands who subjected 184 studies that evaluated 218 diagnostic tests to a critical review.[15] The *diagnostic odds ratio (DOR)*, a measure similar to the likelihood ratio that compares the odds of a positive test result in a person with disease to the odds of a positive result in someone without disease, was computed for each study. DORs were then compared for studies that employed case-control designs to evaluate diagnostic tests and those that utilized broader clinical populations. The worry was that case-control studies frequently utilize sicker, hospitalized subjects and omit cases of milder illness (the spectrum of disease). This phenomenon could create an overestimate of both sensitivity and specificity. Sure enough, the *relative diagnostic odds ratios* were much higher for case-control designs than for those that used a more general population. In other words, the diagnostic accuracy of tests was overestimated when case-control designs were utilized and the spectrum of disease was limited.

Patient referral and selection patterns may also influence test characteristics. Researchers from Los Angeles were surprised by the apparent decline, over several years of use in their institution, in specificity of exercise radionuclide ventriculography as an aid to diagnosing coronary artery disease.[16] To clarify these impressions, they analyzed the results of ventriculography among 77 angiographically normal patients during 2 consecutive periods of time. Patients evaluated in the first 2-year period had a high proportion of normal responses (80–90% specificity) for the test. Patients evaluated during the later 3 years demonstrated normal responses only 35–50% of the time. One explanation for these results recalls the recurrent theme of selection bias. The investigators found that patients in the early group were a healthier sample than those tested later on. The subjects were younger, had less angina, and could endure bicycle exercise longer. When risk factors were combined, the pretest probability of coronary artery disease was 5 times higher for patients who were tested later. The sobering conclusion was that "sicker patients" have a higher rate of abnormal ventriculography responses even though the "gold standard" of angiography is "normal." The authors also note a second factor that appeared to contribute to the declining specificity of the test. They found that confidence in the accuracy of radionuclide ventriculography had prompted clinicians to schedule the test *prior* to performance of angiography. Patients with abnormal ventriculography became preferentially selected for referral for angiograms during the late time period. Early on, angiography preceded ventriculography in most cases. Changes in test sequencing over time and consequent changes in the selection of patients who received both diagnostic procedures appeared to influence the assessment of the accuracy of ventriculography.

STANDARDS

To this point we have devoted our discussion to the diagnostic tests or clinical signs being evaluated, but we have paid little mind to the standards against which tests are compared. We have taken for granted that we really knew who had prostate cancer or bacteremia. How do we know who truly has disease and who does not? Are the standards against which we measure tests valid? The answer depends on which standard we use, since standards vary widely. Sometimes biopsy and histologic examination are utilized, other times serology; still other tests are validated by combinations of clinical impressions and laboratory or radiologic determinations. It should be remembered that all these methods have their own limitations and rates of error. Pathologists can misinterpret histologic sections, serologic tests may in themselves lack sufficient sensitivity to uniformly detect disease, and clinical impressions are woefully susceptible to observer error.

Familiar principles from previous chapters should rattle in our ears. Standards are diagnostic end points and—like entry criteria, treatment descriptions, and other determinations of outcome—must be clearly and satisfactorily defined. Biases can be introduced by observers who know of the test results before they read histologic sections or count colonies on the confirming culture. Conversely, knowledge of the true diagnosis may influence the interpretation of radiologic scans or findings on physical examination. Watch for these. Test results may affect the rigor with which standards are applied. When a test is positive, clinicians will look harder to find disease than when results are negative. More tests are ordered, additional x-rays are obtained, exploratory surgery is undertaken. Standards are unevenly applied. Often this cannot be avoided, since it is difficult to subject patients to invasive and expensive procedures without some justification.

Evaluations of screening programs for breast and prostate cancer are hampered by the uneven assessment of truth brought about by a *verification* or *workup bias*. When mammograms or prostate-specific antigen (PSA) assays are used to screen, the "truth" is determined by biopsy. Individuals with suspicious lesions will have histologic diagnoses made. True positives and false positives can be reasonably estimated. We will have a good idea of the test's predictive value. Valid estimates of sensitivity will be much less satisfactory. Those for whom mammography or PSA assay is negative do not have biopsies unless some other tests hint at the presence of a lesion. Yet some undetected cancers are certain to exist. These will be false negatives that will go unappreciated because we are unable to apply our standard uniformly. Even when alternative tests turn up cancers that screening fails to find, our best guess of sensitivity will remain an overestimate.

For many diseases, a single valid standard is not available. Take heart attack, for example. Without evidence of coronary occlusion and tissue death, the diagnosis of myocardial infarction must be made on a combination of clinical and laboratory features. Most clinicians rely on history of chest pain, evidence of disturbed myocardial rhythm or function, the results of the electrocardiogram, and a variety of serum-enzyme determinations to make the decision whether or not a patient has had a heart attack. While using a combination of clinical and laboratory observations is a perfectly legitimate diagnostic technique, it is not permissible to use the results of the test being evaluated as part of the standard. Surprisingly enough, this has been done. Studies have described the utility of particular muscle enzyme patterns in predicting myocardial infarction and have included, in the criteria for truth, clinical impressions that incorporate the enzyme results. It is not surprising to find reasonably good sensitivity for a test that is both predictor and standard.

SUMMARY

Sensitivity, specificity, and predictive value are tools clinicians can use to evaluate the cornucopia of diagnostic offerings described in medical journals. In the final analysis, the reader must decide whether taking on a new test is beneficial. Clinical benefits must be weighed against medical risks and financial liabilities. Do blood cultures really improve the ability to identify seriously ill children? Do the costs of performing MRI on patients with headaches pay off? Does the poor specificity of mammography, which results in biopsy of many women without malignant breast disease, negate its value as a diagnostic test? These are difficult questions, but it is essential that every new diagnostic test undergoes rigorous scrutiny. If the test does not do it better or less expensively, it is not worth using.

When articles offer information on new diagnostic tests, new applications of old tests, or novel ways of utilizing clinical symptoms and signs to identify diseases, ask the following questions:

1. Have sensitivity, specificity, and predictive values been calculated? Do the authors give evidence that they understand the importance of misclassifying patients into disease (false-positive) or nondisease (false-negative) categories? Has predictive value been correctly ascertained with reference to the prevalence of the disease in the population?

2. Has the problem of spectrum been considered? Do subjects on whom a test's sensitivity and specificity are being determined have severe or late-stage manifestations of disease? Are the results of tests on these individuals likely to apply to subjects who are less ill?

3. Is a reasonable standard being used? Are the histologic-serologic or clinical impressions being used to measure the test's validity reasonable proxies of truth? Have standards been applied equally

to all patients in the evaluation? If not everyone has had an x-ray or blood test, have patients who truly have disease been missed? Have authors avoided the temptation to include the test being evaluated as part of the standard? Have they guarded against bias by keeping standard evaluators protected from the influence of knowing test results?

4. Does the test improve on the present state of affairs? Is it more accurate, less costly, less painful, less time consuming, or in some other way better than the diagnostic techniques currently in practice?

REFERENCES

1. McGowan JE Jr et al: Bacteremia in febrile children seen in a "walk-in" pediatric clinic. N Engl J Med 1973;288:1309.
2. Casscells W, Schoenberger A, Graboys TB: Interpretation by physicians of clinical laboratory results. N Engl J Med 1978;299:999.
3. Cleary PD et al: Compulsory premarital screening for the human immunodeficiency virus: Technical and public health considerations. JAMA 1987;258:1757.
4. Turnock BJ, Kelly CJ: Mandatory premarital testing for human immunodeficiency virus. JAMA 1989;261:3415.
5. Bergman AB, Stamm SJ: The morbidity of cardiac non-disease in schoolchildren. N Engl J Med 1967;276:1008.
6. Elmore JG et al: Ten-year risk of false positive screening mammograms and clinical breast examinations. N Engl J Med 1998;338(16):1089.
7. Wagner JM, McKinney WP, Carpenter JL: Does this patient have appendicitis? JAMA 1996;276(19):1589.
8. Lydick E et al: Development and validation of a simple questionnaire to facilitate identification of women likely to have low bone density. Am J Manag Care 1998;4(1):37.
9. Lemeshow S et al: A method for predicting survival and mortality of ICU patients using objectively derived weights. Crit Care Med 1985;13:519.
10. Poses RM et al: The importance of disease prevalence in transporting clinical prediction rules. Ann Intern Med 1986;105:586.
11. Von Muhlen D et al: Evaluation of the simple calculated osteoporosis risk estimation (SCORE) in older Caucasian women: The Rancho Bernardo study. Osteoporos Int 1999;10(1):79.
12. Ransohoff DF, Feinstein AR: Problems of spectrum and bias in evaluating the efficacy of diagnostic tests. N Engl J Med 1978;299:926.

13. Foti AG et al: Detection of prostatic cancer by solid-phase radioimmunoassay of serum prostatic acid phosphatase. N Engl J Med 1977;297:1357.
14. Fletcher RH: Carcinoembryonic antigen. Ann Intern Med 1986;104:66.
15. Lijmer JG et al: Empirical evidence of design-related bias in studies of diagnostic tests. JAMA 1999;282(11):1061.
16. Rozanski A et al: The declining specificity of exercise radionuclide ventriculography. N Engl J Med 1983;309:518.

Interpretation: Risk

Beware the jabberwock, my son!
The jaws that bite, the claws that catch!
Beware the Jubjub bird, and shun
The frumious Bandersnatch!

LEWIS CARROLL, *THROUGH THE LOOKING-GLASS*

Risks lurk everywhere. If you have asthma, inhaling pollutants puts you at risk of exacerbation. Placing a foot down on the accelerator pedal of your Porsche increases your risk of automotive mortality. Consuming nitrite preservatives and food dyes may predispose you to cancer. Simply belonging to a family in which heart disease or diabetes prevails can increase your chances of developing these diseases later in life. Taking medication to reduce your risk of osteoporosis may increase the likelihood of a blood clot.

Clinicians are faced with scores of implicit risks each day. They must constantly balance the benefits of treatment plans against potential liabilities. How likely is a 21-year-old primigravida with elevated blood pressure and proteinuria to develop eclampsia at delivery? What is the probability that a child with a febrile convulsion will develop epilepsy? What do you tell a 49-year-old with angina about chances of surviving bypass surgery? Should a postmenopausal woman be given estrogen replacement therapy? Although the numbers are not always there to quantify the choices, the use of risk to weigh therapeutic choices and estimate future events occurs constantly in the clinical setting.

Risk serves several additional purposes in journal articles. Researchers use comparative risks to unravel the etiology of diseases, such as multiple sclerosis and breast cancer, or to demonstrate the effectiveness of interventions such as vaccination or isoniazid prophylaxis in preventing polio and tuberculosis. Public health planners gauge the risks of sexually transmitted diseases or drug abuse among subgroups of our population in order to focus their intervention efforts.

In this chapter we will examine the concept of risk as it is presented in medical journals and try to make a potential Jabberwock less intimidating.

EXPRESSING STATEMENTS OF RISK

Basic risk statements express the likelihood that a particular event will occur within a particular population. For example, they indicate the number of cases of rhabdomyolysis among patients taking statin drugs or the frequency with which Down syndrome will occur in babies born to women over 40 years old. The virtue of the basic risk statement lies with its denominator: the number of people at risk. All too often when we read of medical events, we learn only of the numerator—that is, of the patients who developed the rhabdomyolysis or who came down with toxic shock syndrome. Knowing the denominator helps—for example, the number of patients taking statins or women using tampons. Risk statements are proportions that keep medical adversities in their place. We will consider several approaches to describing risk—using ratios and differences. Each has its contribution to make.

Risk Ratios

In conveying ideas about risk, we attempt to isolate specific exposures or behaviors that we believe may be responsible for an illness or other health-related outcome. Alternatively, we wish to convey the size of a benefit provided by an intervention. A logical approach is to compare some measure of disease occurrence among those with and those without the exposure or intervention of interest. How much more likely are those occupationally exposed to benzene to develop leukemia than those not exposed? How much less likely to develop heart disease are those prescribed a statin for high cholesterol levels than those in a placebo group? Such comparisons are readily accomplished by constructing a ratio. When data are collected in a follow-up fashion (whether observational or experimental) and we know the number of cases that develop in each group over a period of time, we have rates that can be compared. The terminology implied to describe this activity travels under several aliases. Readers will find references to *relative risk, risk ratio*, and *rate ratio. Relative risk* is used generally to define the proportion that compares disease occurrences in exposed individuals with those unexposed.

Risk and rate ratios are relative risk statements with shadings of denominator difference. *Risk ratios* describe new cases of an illness or outcome that occur in a fixed cohort or population during a specified period of time. *Rate ratios* have the same cumulative new cases, but rather than utilizing a fixed cohort as the denominator, accept the inflows and outflows of subjects in a population. We encountered this concept earlier as *person-years of observation.* One subject may be followed up for 1 year, another for 5, and each contributes a different number of person-years to the denominator when rates are calculated. Many authors make little distinction between calculations of risk and rate in constructing their ratios. And, for the most part, the distinction is of little practical importance. The general notion is that relative risk is a measure of the strength of the association between a particular exposure (risk factor) or intervention and an outcome. The larger the risk or rate ratio, the stronger the association. Let us look at a few examples of how ratios of risk are employed.

Episodes of meningococcal disease that break out on college campuses always attract media attention. Alarm is considerable and the question is often asked why a population of healthy young adults seems so susceptible to this serious disease. A team headed by investigators from the Centers for Disease Control and Prevention (CDC) used national surveillance data to identify risk factors associated with meningococcal disease among college students.[1] Their numerators consisted of all the cases of meningococcal disease reported by state health departments to the national center over 1 year. Denominators for the risk estimates came primarily from statistics collected by the Department of Education. Table 11–1 shows rates of meningococcal disease among college students sorted by several student characteristics. Ratios can be easily computed by creating proportions of rates of those with and without the characteristics. For example, it becomes readily

TABLE 11–1

Rates of meningococcal disease in college students, September 1998 to August 1999

Characteristic	No. of cases	Population (× 1,000,000)	Rates per 100,000 (95% confidence interval)
18-23 years, nonstudents	211	14.6	1.4 (1.3-1.7)
All college students	96	14.9	0.6 (0.5-0.8)
Undergraduates	93	12.8	0.7 (0.6-0.9)
Freshmen	44	2.3	1.9 (1.4-2.6)
Nonfreshmen	52	12.6	0.4 (0.3-0.5)
Dormitory resident	48	2.1	2.3 (1.7-3.1)
Freshmen in dormitories	30	0.6	5.1 (3.4-7.2)
Male	50	6.6	0.8 (0.6-1.0)
Female	46	8.3	0.6 (0.4-0.7)
White	86	10.6	0.8 (0.6-1.0)
Black	3	1.6	0.2 (0.04-0.6)

Modified, with permission, from Bruce et al.[1]

apparent that college students have a lower risk of contracting meningo-coccal disease than nonstudents of a comparable age. Their rate of 0.6 per 100,000 compared with the 1.4 per 100,000 rate among nonstudents yields a ratio of .43, substantially less than 1. However, among college students, there are increased risks associated with being a freshman, being male, and being White. The greatest increased risk comes with being a freshman (4.7 times as likely to contract meningococcal disease as a nonfreshman); being White carries with it a fourfold increased risk, while being a male has a ratio of 1.3, a 30% increase. For meningococcal disease, coming to live in a new environment in close proximity to others is risky business.

Statements of relative risk do not always bring bad news, however. Recall the cohort study that related walking to protection from cardiovascular disease mortality.[2] In this study adverse outcomes were inversely related to the amount and pace of walking. As seen in Table 11–2, relative risks are less than 1 (indicating protection rather than adverse risk) and decline further as levels of exercise increase. At the most vigorous levels of activity, the risk of heart disease is only 50% of that for nonactive subjects. Exercise is a risk that is well worth taking.

TABLE 11-2

Distribution of indicators of coronary risk and outcomes according to quintile group for total physical-activity score at baseline and relative risk of coronary events

Variable	Quintile group for total physical activity[a]				
	1	2	3	4	5
No. of women	13,859	15,065	14,598	14,326	14,640
Total physical activity score (MET-hour/week)					
Median	0.8	3.2	7.7	15.4	35.4
	Percentage of group				
Risk indicator					
Currently smoking	28.2	23.7	19.6	17.4	17.5
History of hypertension	26.1	25.1	24.0	22.4	21.0
History of diabetes	4.2	3.3	3.7	2.8	2.6
History of hypercholesterolemia	12.0	11.4	11.7	11.6	10.6
Current postmenopausal hormone replacement therapy	19.5	21.5	23.1	23.8	24.1
Use of multivitamin supplement	36.9	39.9	43.0	45.0	47.2
	Mean				
Age, years	52.1	52.3	52.2	52.2	52.3
Alcohol consumption (g/day)	5.9	5.8	6.0	6.4	7.0
Body mass index	25.1	24.6	24.2	23.9	23.5
	Outcomes				
No. of coronary events	178	153	124	101	89
Person-year of follow-up	106,252	116,175	112,703	110,886	113,419
	Relative risk				
Type of analysis					
Age-adjusted	1.0	0.77	0.65	0.54	0.46
Multivariate[b]	1.0	0.88	0.81	0.74	0.66

[a]The total physical activity score was expressed as MET-hours per week, calculated as the average time per week spent in each of 8 activities; multiplied by the MET value of each activity. The MET value is the caloric needs during exercise divided by the caloric needs at rest.
[b]The model included variables for age (in 5-year categories), period during the study (four 2-year periods), smoking status (never smoked, previously smoked, or currently smokes 1-14, 15-24, or ≥25 cigarettes per day), body mass index (in 5 categories), menopausal status (premenopausal, postmenopausal without hormone replacement therapy, postmenopausal with previous hormone replacement therapy, or postmenopausal with current hormone replacement therapy), parental history with respect to myocardial infarction before the age of 60 years, multivitamin supplement use, vitamin E supplement use, alcohol consumption (0, 1-4, 5-14, or ≥15 g/day), history of hypertension, history of diabetes, history of hypercholesterolemia, and aspirin use (none, 1-6 doses per week, or 7 or more doses per week).
Modified, with permission, from Manson et al.[2]

Investigators who were looking for factors that would predict survival of patients who were discharged from a coronary care unit discovered that the support offered by "animal companions" provided protection from mortality.[3] Ninety-two men and women who were recovering from heart attacks or bouts of angina pectoris supplied information on a broad range of personal topics, including pet ownership. A year after hospitalization, follow-up was done to discover the status of the patients. Fourteen of the 92 patients had died. When death rates were calculated according to pet ownership, only 3 of 53 pet owners (5.6%) were no longer living, compared with 11 of 39 (28%) patients who were without animal companions. The relative risk of 5.6 per 100 ÷ 28 per 100, or 0.2, means only one-fifth the mortality, or a fivefold greater likelihood of survival, if one has a furry or a feathered friend. That is an impressive difference! Perhaps prescriptions for beagles rather than beta-blockers should be offered at discharge from coronary care units.

The large randomized trial known as the Women's Health Initiative (WHI) provides a selection of risk statements in an effort to summarize the benefits and liabilities of hormone replacement therapy (HRT).[4] At the time the trial was designed, HRT was thought to be helpful in protecting women from coronary heart disease (CHD) and hip fracture due to osteoporosis. Over 16,000 postmenopausal women with uteri intact between the ages of 50 and 79 years were randomly assigned to receive an estrogen-progestin combination pill or placebo. Although the trial was scheduled to continue for 8 years, it was terminated after only 5 when it became apparent that the risks of HRT were outweighing benefits. A tally appears in Table 11–3. The bad news certainly appears to exceed the good. Adverse risk ratios include those for CHD, stroke, breast cancer, and pulmonary embolism. Only risks from hip fracture and colorectal cancer are less than unity and suggest benefit. To assist in the overall assessment of the medication, the investigators construct a "global index" consisting of the major risk factors noted above, plus endometrial cancer and mortality from other causes. This composite risk turns out to be 1.15 (95% CI, 1.03-1.28), indicating net harm from using HRT as a disease preventative.

Relative Risk & Study Design

When we start with a population, as we do in follow-up studies, the calculation of relative risk is straightforward. We know in advance who eats

TABLE 11-3

Risk of clinical outcomes for women taking estrogen plus progestin (E+P) or placebo for an average of 5.2 years in the Women's Health Initiative

| Outcome | No. of subjects | | Risk ratio | %change | Risk difference per 10,000/year |
	E+P n=8506	Placebo n=8102			
Coronary heart disease	164	122	1.29	29	7
Stroke	127	85	1.41	41	8
Pulmonary embolism	70	31	2.13	113	8
Breast cancer	166	124	1.26	26	8
Colorectal cancer	45	67	0.63	-37	-6
Hip fracture	44	62	0.66	-34	-5
Global index[a]	751	623	1.15	15	19

[a]Global index = Any of six events listed or endometrial cancer or any death due to other causes.
Based on Rossouw et. al.(4)

carrots and who does not. We classify these people and remeasure them later to see who has developed poor eyesight. Table 11–4 illustrates how relative risk is created when a population with known risk-factor status is observed.

Case-control studies are trickier. Since the design enlists patients who already have poor vision, sorts them according to who consumes carrots, and makes the comparison with an independently selected control group, a common population base is lacking. The true risk of disease cannot be calculated. We need to know about the relative rates of developing bad eyesight, not the relative rates of carrot eating. The problem is depicted in Table 11–5. We cannot move horizontally across the table to develop rates of disease for persons with and without a particular factor. The expression "$A/(A + B)/C/(C + D),$" which would give us the relative risk, cannot be calculated because the cases and controls are not represented in relation to their prevalence in any parent population.

However, there are ways of estimating relative risk from the case-control design. By tolerating two assumptions, we can come up with a

		TABLE 11–4	
		Relative risk in population-based (follow-up) studies	

	Disease present	Disease absent	
Factor present	A	B	$A + B$
Factor absent	C	D	$C + D$

$$\text{Relative risk} = \frac{\text{rate of disease in people with factor}}{\text{rate of disease in people without factor}}$$

$$= \frac{\text{disease present/people with factor}}{\text{disease present/people without factor}}$$

$$= \frac{A/(A+B)}{C/(C+D)}$$

$$\text{Disease prevalence} = \frac{A+C}{A+B+C+D)}$$

serviceable substitute. First, we must hope that the control group is reasonably representative of the general population with respect to the occurrence of risk factors. Then, if the disease is relatively uncommon (as is true with most noninfectious diseases), A and C in Table 11–5 will be quite small in comparison with B and D. If we simply use B and D as approximations for $A + B$ and $C + D$, respectively, the problem of disease frequency no longer interferes with our calculations. The estimate of relative risk can be expressed as $A/B/C/D$ or, in simplified form, AD/BC. This *cross-product* estimate of relative risk is referred to as the *relative odds,* or *odds ratio.* (A/B and C/D represent *odds,* the ratio of those with risk factor to those without the factor among cases and controls, respectively.) Purists are careful not to call this calculation a true relative risk, since the individual risk rates are approximations only.

In an effort to find more about possible risk factors for meningococcal disease, the investigators who studied the problem among college students

TABLE 11–5
Relative risk estimate in case-control studies

	Cases	Controls	
Factor present	A	B	$A + B$
Factor absent	C	D	$C + D$

Relative risk $=$ $\dfrac{\text{rate of disease in people with factor}}{\text{rate of disease in people without factor}}$

But . . . $\dfrac{E}{A + B}$ and $\dfrac{C}{C + D}$ do not represent rate of disease in a population

If . . . disease has a low frequency, so that A and C are small relative to B and D in the population at large

Then . . . $\dfrac{A}{B}$ approximates $\dfrac{A}{A + B}$

and

$\dfrac{C}{D}$ approximates $\dfrac{C}{C + D}$

And . . . relative risk is approximated by $\dfrac{A / B}{C / D}$ or $\dfrac{A \times D}{B \times C}$

conducted a case-control study within their larger population-based effort.[1] They identified a group of 50 meningococcal disease patients and then selected 3 control subjects for each patient, matched for college, sex, and undergraduate versus graduate status. Table 11–6 displays a collection of risk factors that were assessed, the number and percentage of cases and controls reporting the factor, and the odds ratio obtained. The odds ratios were similar to the relative risks we observed earlier. Being White, a freshman, and living in a dormitory are the strongest predictors of developing disease. Consuming alcoholic beverages, attending parties, and kissing

TABLE 11-6
Risk factors for meningococcal disease

Risk factor	Case-patients No. (%) (N = 50)	Controls No. (%) (n = 148)	Matched OR (95% CI)	P value
Freshman	26 (52)	38 (26)	3.0 (1.6-5.9)	.001
Freshman in dormitory	23 (46)	28 (19)	3.7 (1.8-7.7)	.001
Dormitory residence	33 (66)	67 (45)	2.7 (1.3-5.6)	.008
Consumed ≥ 5 alcoholic drinks[a]	26 (52)	50 (34)	2.4 (1.2-4.9)	.02
Frequented ≥ 3 parties or bars[a]	19 (38)	36 (24)	2.2 (1.0-4.7)	.04
Kissed ≥ 2 persons on the mouth[b]	17 (34)	28 (19)	2.3 (1.1-4.8)	.03
White race	48 (96)	120 (82)	5.4 (1.2-24.2)	.03
Attended ≥ 1 movie	30 (61)	117 (79)	0.4 (0.2-0.9)	.02
Employed during school	17 (34)	74 (50)	0.5 (0.3-0.98)	.04
Active smoking	7 (14)	15 (10)	1.5 (0.5-4.0)	.45

[a]Per week in month of interest.
[b]In month prior to illness.
OR, odds ratio; CI, confidence interval.
Modified, with permission, from Bruce et al.[1]

multiple persons are social acts that also enhance risk. Going to movies and working appear protective (odds ratios less than 1).

Recalling earlier discussions of sampling and inference, it should be clear that odds ratios determined from case-control studies are based on limited samples and are particularly subject to sampling error. Knowledgeable investigators recognize that their data supply only a single estimate of the true relative odds or relative risk. On the basis of their particular findings, they can calculate a range in which the true estimate is likely to fall by constructing a confidence interval (CI) for the risk estimate. It is worth observing that some of the CIs surrounding the estimated odds ratios for meningococcal risk factors are rather wide. The risk factor of White race, for example, with its estimated risk of 5.4 (a rather hefty relative risk) is consistent with a risk range from as low as 1.2 to as high as 24.2. The CI does not include 1 (no additional risk), but a CI this broad should temper our enthusiasm for the result.

RISK DIFFERENCES

Implicit in the process of identifying and defining risk factors is the hope that somehow, by modifying or eliminating risk, health can be improved. How many lives could be saved if seat belts were used more? How much would morbidity be reduced by bringing everyone's blood pressure under control? What impact do we have on the incidence of neonatal infections with a national hepatitis B immunization campaign? Comparison of risks is useful in assessing healthcare prevention and treatment programs; but where causation is best suggested by *ratios* of risks, health impact is addressed by examining the *differences* in risk rates. The *attributable* risk tells us the difference in rates between people who smoke, have high blood pressure, or have susceptibility to hepatitis B and those who do not. It indicates how much of the morbidity or mortality of a disease can be attributed to the risk factor. Attributable risk quantifies the contribution risk factors make in producing disease within a population. By comparing attributable risk for different factors, we can begin to arrange informed healthcare priorities.

Mortality data from the classic study of British doctors' smoking habits demonstrate the difference between relative risk and attributable risk, as Table 11–7 shows.[5] The relative risk of lung cancer caused by smoking is much greater at 32 than is the relative risk of myocardial infarction (MI) among smokers, which is only 1.4. However, heart disease is much more common than lung cancer. Thus, even though the relative risk associated with heart disease and smoking is small, its importance to the general health is magnified. The death rate from heart disease that can be attributed to smoking comes close to that contributed by smoking-induced lung cancer. If cigarette smoking could be eliminated, almost as many deaths from coronary artery disease could be prevented as from lung cancer.

	TABLE 11-7	
Relative risk and attributable risk of cigarette smoking for lung cancer and heart disease		
	Death rate (per 100,000 population)	
	From lung cancer	From coronary disease
For heavy smokers	223	516
For nonsmokers	7	361
Relative risk	$\dfrac{223}{7} = 32$	$\dfrac{516}{361} = 1.4$
Attributable risk	$223 - 7 = 216$	$516 - 361 = 155$

Modified, with permission, from Doll and Hill.[5]

Evaluations of interventions also use risk differences to express benefits (and liabilities). A large multicenter randomized trial evaluated the benefits of raloxifene hydrochloride (a selective estrogen receptor modulator, or SERM) on the risk of vertebral fractures in postmenopausal women with osteoporosis.[6] This elegant study enrolled 77,000 women in 25 countries. Subjects had been postmenopausal for at least 2 years and all had osteoporosis according to bone mineral density criteria developed by the World Health Organization. In addition, about one-third of the subjects had at least one preexisting vertebral fracture. Women were randomly allocated to 1 of 3 groups—placebo, raloxifene at 60 mg/day, or raloxifene at 120 mg/day. They were followed up for 3 years and assessed periodically with radiographs of the spine.

Results of the study can be seen in Table 11–8. The risk of fracture (expressed as percentage with new fractures) drops in the raloxifene-treated women. Relative risks among the treated women range from about 0.5 to 0.7 with CIs all well below 1, indicating protection. Risk differences vary between the groups of women who were with and without fractures at enrollment. Subjects without previous fractures lowered their risks of new fractures (from 4.5 to 2.8% for the higher drug dosage). Women with existing fractures had a much higher risk of new fracture (21.2%), which fell to 10.7% with treatment. Consequently, the reduction in fracture risk among these women attributable to raloxifene, while comparable in relative terms, has a substantially larger difference. Almost 10 of

TABLE 11-8

New vertebral fracture (VF) in 6828 postmenopausal women receiving placebo or raloxifene hydrochloride therapy for osteoporosis

	Placebo	Raloxifene 60 mg/day	Raloxifene 120 mg/day
Low bone density			
No. of women	1522	1490	1512
Women with ≥ 1 VF (%)	68 (4.5)	35 (2.3)	42 (2.8)
RR (95% CI)	...	0.5 (0.4-0.8)	0.5 (0.4-0.9)
No. of women needed to treat[a]	...	46	59
Low bone density + prevalent VF			
No. of women	770	769	765
Women with ≥ 1 VF (%)	163 (21.2)	113 (14.7)	82 (10.7)
RR (95% CI)	...	0.7 (0.6-0.9)	0.5 (0.4-0.7)
No. of women needed to treat[a]	...	16	10

[a]For 3 years to prevent 1 incident of vertebral fracture.
RR, relative risk; CI, confidence interval.
Modified, with permission, from Ettinger et al.[6]

every 100 women with previous fractures who took the higher-dose raloxifene were spared new fractures compared with only 2 per 100 in the group without prior fractures.

To make this information more meaningful to clinicians, the authors present the data as the *number needed to treat* (Table 11–8). This is calculated by taking the reciprocal of the risk difference between placebo and raloxifene-treated subjects, that is, 1 divided by the risk difference. The number tells us how many subjects must receive the treatment to avoid 1 adverse outcome (in this case, vertebral fracture). Comparisons are easy. Incorporated in the calculation are not only risk differences but also the magnitude of the baseline risk itself. Women in the raloxifene study who entered with a preexisting fracture were at almost fivefold greater risk than those without fractures (21.2% ÷ 4.5%). That increased risk is reflected in the fewer numbers needed to treat to prevent each new fracture (16 and 10 compared with 46 and 59).

BALANCING RISKS

Assessing risk differences may give one a different perspective on the estrogen-progestin results from the Women's Health Initiative (WHI). When increased relative risks of 29% for CHD and 26% for invasive breast cancer are announced, there is reason for concern. But risk differences, which include information on *denominators*, that is, the number of women who are taking HRT and are at risk for adverse events might modify one's interpretation (refer to Table 11–2). For every 10,000 women who take HRT for a year we can anticipate 7 CHD events, 8 strokes, 8 pulmonary embolisms, and 8 breast cancers attributable to the medication. Referring to the global index we see that an additional 19 adverse events occur among the women taking HRT. Somehow these numbers seem less daunting than those conveyed by the relative risk. The data still suggest that widespread use of HRT cannot be recommended as a disease prevention measure since thousands of adverse events would result. However, individual women who experience relief from postmenopausal symptoms with HRT might find a rate of 2 in 1000 per year a palatable risk.

Risks & Benefits

The concept of risk helps us identify the perils of our environment and quantify the likelihood of beneficial or adverse medical outcomes. It should guide informed decisions, but we can sometimes lose our perspective. Announcement that a new hair spray has been linked to cancer or that a drug may be a risk factor for birth defects raises an emotional response that occasionally threatens perspective. Balancing risk is important.

Because of the observation that women who smoke cigarettes excrete reduced levels of estrogen in their urine and because of the known link between estrogen and endometrial cancer, a case-control study was conducted to determine whether cigarette smokers might have a reduced incidence of this reproductive tract cancer.[7] A total of 510 women who had invasive endometrial cancer were interviewed for historic information on use of several potential carcinogens. A control group of 727 women who had other malignancies that are thought to be unrelated to cigarette use served as controls. Twenty-nine percent of controls were current smokers, compared with only 22% of endometrial cancer patients. The risk of cancer for smoking women was 0.7, with a 95% CI of 0.5–1.0. For women who smoked 25 cigarettes per day or more, the risk was even lower, at 0.5. This evidence suggests that smoking protects women from developing endometrial cancer, presumably by lowering estrogen secretion.

After all the terrible things we have said about cigarette smoking, here is evidence that the "evil weed" may have beneficial health effects. However, this "benefit" must be put into perspective with the overall adverse risk of tobacco use. The authors themselves are quick to point out that their results should not be interpreted as an endorsement for smoking. In an editorial commentary, Weiss[8] calculates that if smoking turned out to be protective, it would reduce the annual risk of endometrial cancer among postmenopausal women from approximately 100 per 100,000 to 70 per 100,000. On the basis of the mortality rate of the disease, he figures approximately 6 lives per 100,000 smokers would be saved annually. This is certainly not a large number and compares poorly with the lives lost annually because of cigarette smoking, which is estimated to be 30 times as high.[8]

Whenever medical decisions are made, adverse risks must be balanced against the potential benefits of the medication, surgical procedure, or immunization program. In the raloxifene study, the benefits of treatment in reducing vertebral fracture are clear: A reduction in risk of 30–50% was observed. However, there is a downside to the drug. Raloxifene is associated with adverse events. Raloxifene takers experienced significantly more hot flashes, leg cramps, and edema than placebo recipients. They also had a greater risk of venous thromboembolic events (blood clots)— a relative risk of 3.1. One needs to weigh this adverse risk against the benefits of the treatment. It turns out that the *absolute risk* of thromboemboli is low: 0.3% among placebo recipients and 1.0% in each of the raloxifene-treated groups. Analogous to the *number needed to treat,* one can compute a *number needed to harm.* This will be the number of subjects treated for each adverse event to occur. In the case of raloxifene-induced blood clots, the number needed to harm would be 1/(1.0%–0.3%), or 1 patient of every 142 treated. This risk must be placed against the benefits the drug has demonstrated in reducing new vertebral fractures.

But there is more. This investigation, known as the Multiple Outcomes of Raloxifene Evaluation, assessed other clinical outcomes.[6] Included were reductions in *nonvertebral* fractures and development of breast cancer. (Estrogen receptor modulators should lower the risk of breast cancer.) Study results indicated no significant reduction in wrist, ankle, or hip fractures as a result of treatment. However, raloxifene takers had a 70% reduced rate of breast cancer (relative risk, 0.3; 95% CI, 0.2–0.6) compared with placebo, a tantalizing finding that is prompting further investigation.

COSTS & BENEFITS

It is no longer possible to discuss treatment benefits in terms of clinical outcomes alone. Scarcely a journal passes our plates that does not make mention of some economic aspect of health care. Increasing numbers of feature articles appear in journals that address the cost-effectiveness of a medication, surgical procedure, screening program, or service delivery innovation. Many of these studies are quite complex and bring with them a whole new vocabulary: cost-benefit, cost-effectiveness, sensitivity analysis, incremental cost-effectiveness, utilities, and quality-adjusted life-years, to mention a few. The level of sophistication in many of these studies is substantial—well beyond the scope of our present discussion. Some solid resources are available, however.[9,10]

As an appetizer to the topic, let us return to the problem of meningococcal disease in college students. The high risk of developing disease in subgroups of the college population and the availability of a meningococcal vaccine suggest preventive strategies. Would implementing an immunization program make sense? What would be the costs of such a program?

A group of public health researchers performed an economic analysis to address these questions.[11] The investigators decided that targeting the group of freshmen who live in dormitories would be a logical place to start as these students have the highest risk of contracting the disease of all the subgroups listed in Table 11–1, 5.1 cases/100,000. There are about 600,000 of such students nationwide of whom 30 can be expected to contract meningococcal meningitis every year. However, calculating the costs and benefits* of immunizing these students is not a simple matter. It requires a number of considerations.

---

*Although we speak broadly of cost-benefit analyses, this term technically refers to comparisons made in strictly monetary terms. Costs are measured in dollars (at least in the United States) and benefits as well. This becomes a problem in many studies because it requires that health outcomes be reduced to monetary values. Many find it difficult or objectionable to attach a price to human illness and death. Most economic analyses that readers will encounter fall under the rubric of cost-effectiveness studies. The cost part of the equation is the same, but "effectiveness" is measured in more human dimensions, such as added years of life or quality of life.

To begin with, the vaccine is not 100% efficacious even in the best of circumstances. Current preparations have most but not all of the bacterial serotypes that may cause disease represented in the product. (About 75% of the serogroups responsible for U.S. epidemics are included in the vaccine.) Nor will everyone given the vaccine have a protective immunologic response. (Estimates of vaccine efficacy range from 80 to 95%.) Not everyone eligible for vaccine will receive it. Some will refuse; others will be unavailable.

In analyzing the economics, one needs to determine the net of expenses and savings that will result from the program. Costs will be incurred in purchasing doses of vaccine and in paying people to corral students and administer the vaccine. There may also be adverse effects of the vaccine that result in medical care expenses, including outpatient visits and even hospitalizations. On the positive side, a successful vaccination program will reduce the healthcare costs of treating meningococcal illness. One can also factor in as a saving the value of a premature death based on an estimate of what that individual's lifetime productivity might have been, or lost productivity due to long-term disability in the wake of the disease. One could spin a considerably more elaborate web that includes costs to the family of visiting an ill son or daughter, lost work productivity associated with the illness, and so forth. A comprehensive list of all the possible economic implications of an illness can be extensive. The present example limits considerations to those that are most obvious.

Economic evaluations rest on a number of assumptions. Estimates of vaccine efficacy, coverage of the target population, cost of administration, and healthcare costs are all subject to variation. To account for this, investigators often perform a *sensitivity analysis*. This means that as they go through their calculations, they use a range of estimates for each of the critical components. This in turn produces a range of estimates for the final product, some boundaries (not unlike the confidence interval) within which we can expect our answer to lie.

For the CDC analysis, the range of estimates can be seen in Table 11–9. The strategy of vaccinating the high-risk group of freshmen living in dormitories would require approximately 350,000–590,000 doses of vaccine annually. It would prevent only 15–30 cases of meningococcal disease and 1–3 deaths over a 4-year interval. The cost per case prevented under this option would be $600,000–$1.9 million, with a cost for each death prevented of $7 million to $20 million. These costs are high. Whether they are worth the program benefits becomes a policy rather than a medical

TABLE 11-9
Valuations of benefits[a] and costs[b] of meningococcal vaccination program for first-year college students living in dormitories

Variable	Range of values ($/student)
Benefits	
Hospital care per case	10,924-24,030
Value of life lost (in productivity)	1.2-4.8 million
Treatment of sequelae	1298-14,600
Costs	
Vaccine and administration	54-88
Treatment of vaccine side effects	7000-24,540 (per million doses)

[a]The savings associated with cases and deaths averted.
[b]Costs associated with vaccination.
Modified, with permission, from Scott et al.[11]

question. The authors suggest that "given the low incidence of the disease and the high cost of a vaccination program, scarce public health resources could be targeted to more common health conditions."[11]

Another instructive example of cost-effectiveness analysis comes from the literature on beta-blockers.[12] We noted back in Chapter 5 that beta-blockers, such as timolol, prevent further cardiac events among heart attack survivors. Unfortunately, despite confirmation of these benefits in several well-executed randomized trials, use of the medication in practice has been less than universal. Surveys indicating substantial underuse of beta-blockers prompted investigators to employ existing research data to evaluate health and economic benefits of increasing use of the treatment.[12] They utilized a computer model to simulate two cohorts of subjects: one, a group of patients discharged from the hospital after their first heart attack who were followed up for 20 years; second, a cumulative or multicohort consisting of 20 successive annual cohorts of myocardial infarction survivors. Included in the analysis were a host of variables related to the costs and effectiveness of using beta-blockers after heart attack. Estimated values for these are seen in Table 11–10.

The authors estimate that 92% of MI subjects will be eligible for beta-blocker therapy and that presently only 44% are being treated. Some patients will withdraw from therapy because of complications or adverse events and do not benefit; these are factored into the model. Benefits from

TABLE 11–10

Summary of variables for benefits of beta-blocker use following MI

Variable	Best estimate	Range for sensitivity analyses
Beta-blocker eligibility	92%	60% (upper limit NA)
Beta-blocker use rates	44%	59% (lower limit NA)
Withdrawal rates		
Among patients with no relative contraindications	12%	NA
Among patients with relative contraindications	30%	50% (lower limit NA)
CHD event rate reductions with beta-blocker use		
Myocardial infarction	27%	NA
Sudden death from cardiac arrest	32%	NA
Mortality	22%	NA
Effectiveness	3 years full benefits, then 3 years reduced (7%), then 1% benefits for 14 years	3, 6, or 20 years full benefits
QALY reductions due to beta-blockers	0%	1% for 3 years (lower limit NA)
Beta-blocker costs		
Per person per year	$432	$52–$600
Years of costs	20	6 only (upper limit NA)
Discount rate	3%	0–10%

NA, not applicable; QALY, quality-adjusted life-year; MI, myocardial infarction; CHD, coronary heart disease.
Modified, with permission, from Phillips et al.[12]

treatment include reductions of future MIs and cardiac-induced mortality. Costs per person per year are calculated for the drug. (The analysis does not account for costs associated with adverse drug events, which the authors say would not be significant.) The savings that come from cardiac-related events that do not occur and mortality averted by expanding beta-blocker treatment are used to offset drug costs.

Model results are impressive. Under the single-cohort scenario, 20 years of treatment would result in 4300 fewer coronary deaths, 3500 fewer MIs, and the addition of 45,000 life-years to the population. There would, of course, be a cost to this, which the authors calculate at $4500 per quality-adjusted life-year (QALY) gained.[*] When the multicohort—20 successive years of treatment—is used in the analysis, results are even more impressive. Increasing beta-blocker use could prevent 62,000 MIs and 72,000 coronary heart disease deaths. Over time, bringing usage up to target levels would actually produce cost savings.

A vocabulary travels along with economic analyses. Essential to a good study is the *sensitivity analysis,* in which the assumptions, such as patient eligibility, duration of treatment effectiveness, and costs of drugs, are varied. If results still appear favorable after less favorable assumptions are included in the model, our confidence in the findings is increased. In the "worst-case scenarios" of this beta-blocker study, the costs of treatment increased to $10,000 for each QALY gained, a figure that compares quite favorably with a general notion that amounts less than $40,000 per QALY are cost effective. On the other hand, the authors demonstrate that a moderate reduction in drug costs could push the analysis into positive territory, where increased treatment would actually save money overall.

One bit of economic legerdemain readers encounter is the *discount rate.* The discount rate acknowledges that most people prefer spending money at some time in the future than at the present. Stated another way, given the choice between spending $100 today and $100 10 years from now, most folks would opt for the latter choice. This means that we value present dollars more highly than future dollars. Most economic analyses, therefore, discount the value of future dollars saved or spent to bring all costs or savings in line with current values. Each year into the future, the dollar loses some of its value—generally this is calculated in the range of 3–5%. Again, more thorough explanations are available.[9,10]

---

[*]A *quality-adjusted life-year* (QALY) is a measure of additional survival that incorporates a quality-of-life dimension. Such measures are developed to reflect that survival alone is a crude measure of benefit. The quality of additional years of life may depend on an individual's physical, mental, and social functioning and general life satisfaction. Persistent pain or functional impairment may limit a person's quality of life and is part of the consideration when QALYs are constructed. For a more detailed discussion, see reference 10.

SUMMARY

Statements of risk help us quantify the dangers of the environment; they serve as guides to prognosis and measures of potential effectiveness of health intervention activities. Risk ratios are useful for testing hypotheses about etiologic association. Risk differences provide a population perspective to assess the impact of changing risk factors on health.

Risk statements must be kept in perspective. Estimates of relative risk are derived from samples and, like any other samples, are vulnerable to error. Authors who place confidence intervals around their risk estimates provide readers with helpful information about the true likelihood that a factor is related to disease. Caution must be exercised in interpreting relative risk estimates without information about the absolute magnitude of risk. Risks must be balanced against benefits. Before new treatments are advocated or established medications blacklisted, the overall health impact must be considered.

Economic analyses provide another perspective on risk. They acknowledge that decisions on health expenditures must be made. Readers need to be comfortable with methods of incorporating concepts of costs and benefits into evaluations of care.

REFERENCES

1. Bruce MG et al: Risk factors for meningococcal disease in college students. JAMA 2001;286(6):688.
2. Manson JE et al: A prospective study of walking as compared with vigorous exercise in the prevention of coronary heart disease in women. N Engl J Med 1999;341(9):650.
3. Friedmann E et al: Animal companions and one-year survival after discharge from a coronary care unit. Public Health Rep 1980;95:307.
4. Rossouw J E et al: Risks and benefits of estrogen plus progestin in healthy postmenopausal women: Principal results from the Women's Health Initiative randomized controlled trial. JAMA 2002;288:321.
5. Doll R, Hill AB: Mortality in relation to smoking: Ten years' observations of British doctors. Br Med J 1964;1:1399, 1460.
6. Ettinger B et al: Reduction of vertebral fracture risk in postmenopausal women with osteoporosis treated with raloxifene: Results from a 3-year

randomized clinical trial. Multiple Outcomes of Raloxifene Evaluation (MORE) Investigators. JAMA 1999;282(7):637.

7. Lesko SM et al: Cigarette smoking and the risk of endometrial cancer. N Engl J Med 1985;313:593.
8. Weiss NS: Can not smoking be hazardous to your health? N Engl J Med 1985;313:632.
9. Eisenberg JM: Clinical economics: A guide to the economic analysis of clinical practices JAMA 1989;262:2879.
10. Pettitti DB: *Meta-analysis, Decision Analysis, and Cost-Effectiveness Analysis: Methods for Quantitative Synthesis in Medicine,* 2nd ed. Oxford University Press, 2000.
11. Scott RD II et al: Vaccinating first-year college students living in dormitories for meningococcal disease: An economic analysis. Am J Prev Med 2002;23:98.
12. Phillips KA et al: Health and economic benefits of increased beta-blocker use following myocardial infarction. JAMA 2000;284(21):2748.

CHAPTER TWELVE

Interpretation: Causes

. . . and now remains that we find out the cause of this effect.
Or rather say the cause of this defect. For this effect defective
comes by cause.

HAMLET, ACT II, SCENE II

Poor Polonius, a tracker of truth, trapped in his own logical snares. He never does ferret out the cause of Hamlet's madness. Is it due to unrequited love, a father's death, or Denmark's melancholy climate? Polonius fails to find out. Indeed, he dies midway through the investigation, undone by his own hazardous techniques of study design.

Chasing after causes in medical studies is difficult, though not usually terminal, business. Up to now we have minced about with phrases such as "associated with," "linked to," and "related to." We have avoided dogmatic statements of causation, such as "hormone replacement causes breast cancer" or "air pollution is responsible for increased mortality." We have been reluctant to completely accept that walking wards off heart disease or that birthing rooms are responsible for decreased problems in childbirth. Even when we think we have pinpointed a guilty party, the possibility remains that some unsuspected risk factor is actually causing the disease or an unappreciated cointervention is responsible for the treatment effect. In this chapter, we will look for ways to decide whether the associations found in studies merit consideration as causes, and we will note some ways in which investigators deal with multiple potential explanations for the outcomes they observe.

CONFOUNDING

Spurious appearance of causation can occur through three mechanisms. The first of these is *chance*, where the caprice of sampling variability makes substance out of shadow. The rates of diarrhea caused by azithromycin and amoxicillin-clavulanate appear to be different but, in reality, sample estimates obtained from different portions of a single distribution of side effects create this illusion. We have considered all this in some detail in earlier chapters. *Bias* is the second mechanism. We have seen a variety of ways that spurious results may occur because our selection of comparison subjects is drawn from a sample of people with healthier lifestyles than case subjects or because the stress of illness has caused case subjects to recall their past medical history differently from controls. *Confounding* is the third mechanism.

In Chapter 3, we mentioned confusing or confounding factors in case-control studies. Confounding occurs when factors that relate to both the characteristic under scrutiny and the outcome appear as competing explanations. The example we used was the apparent relationship between cigar smoking and baldness—an association that was confused or confounded by age. The data from this study appear in Table 12–1. We select 50 bald men to represent the cases and find that over one-half of them are cigar smokers. In the control group, only 8 of 50 subjects chosen admit to the habit. Using the cross-product estimation for the odds ratio (OR), we see that there is a sixfold $[(27 \times 42)/(23 \times 8) = 1134/184 = 6.2]$ risk of baldness associated with cigar smoking. However, in examining the data, we realize that the ages of men in the groups being compared are dissimilar. Our bald subjects average 52 years of age, compared with a mean age of 24 years for controls. Quite a disparity! Since we know that increasing age is related both to cigar smoking and to loss of hair, we have a problem with confounding. Matching on age—that is, selecting only control subjects whose age is within several years of the case—is one way of controlling the effects of age. When we redo our study, choosing only cases and controls who are between the ages of 40 and 45 years, the hypothetical results appear as in Table 12–2. Now the rates of cigar

TABLE 12–1

Rate of cigar smoking for bald men compared with controls

		Baldness		
		Yes (cases)	No (controls)	
Cigar smoking	Yes	27	8	
	No	23	42	
		50	50	100

$$\text{Relative odds} = \frac{27 \times 42}{23 \times 8} = \frac{1134}{184} = 6.2$$

smoking are similar for cases and controls, that is, about 40%. The risk ratio, as calculated by the cross-products estimate, is very close to 1. There is no longer an association between smoking and hair loss. Confounding has been eliminated.

Confounding is the epidemiologist's eternal triangle. Any time a risk factor, patient characteristic, or intervention appears to be causing a disease, side effect, or outcome, the relationship needs to be challenged. Are we seeing cause and effect, or is a confounding factor exerting its unappreciated influence? The problem is schematized in Figure 12–1. It is

TABLE 12–2

Rate of cigar smoking for bald men 40–45 years old compared with age-matched controls

		Baldness		
		Yes (cases)	No (controls)	
Cigar smoking	Yes	21	23	
	No	29	27	
		50	50	100

$$\text{Relative odds} = \frac{21 \times 27}{29 \times 23} = \frac{567}{667} = 0.85$$

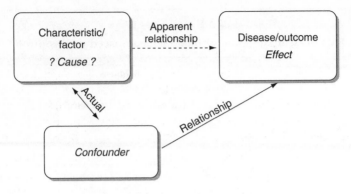

FIGURE 12–1. The confounding triangle.

important to remember that to be a confounding variable, a factor must be related both to the outcome or effect and to the putative cause.

The apparent protective effect that animal companions afforded heart attack victims would seem a situation ripe for confounding.[1] Recall that pet owners had a better than sixfold greater likelihood of survival in the first year following discharge from a coronary care unit than patients who were without animal companions. The authors report that their findings are consistent with the hypothesis that social affiliation and companionship have important, positive health benefits. Are there other equally plausible explanations? Are there other attributes pet owners possess that might contribute to a more favorable outlook for survival after heart attack? Several possibilities come to mind. Perhaps people who tolerate pets possess more easygoing personalities and less coronary-prone, aggressive behavior of the sort that predisposes to future cardiac problems. Perhaps, because pets require attention and care, pet owners tend to be younger and more active than nonowners and thus more likely to survive. Perhaps they walk their animals and get more exercise.

Confounding factors are always lurking, ready to cast doubt on the interpretation of studies. The improved perinatal outcomes of women utilizing the alternative birthing center may not be due to the innovative facility but to the improved outcomes to be expected from the healthier, better educated, more highly motivated volunteers who select the birthing-center option. With confounding a ubiquitous danger, savvy authors will make efforts to deal with these potential alternative explanations.

DEALING WITH CONFOUNDING

Confounding may be attacked either in the design of the study or during analysis. Matching is a technique used in the design stage. Matching, as discussed in Chapter 3, is generally utilized in observational studies. Comparison subjects are selected who share specific similarities (age, weight, race, sex) with the cases. Matched characteristics are eliminated as competing explanations of the disease. Matching before the fact is not always practical. Investigators may not be able to choose ideal controls or may not anticipate potential confounding factors in advance. Techniques are available for controlling the effects of confounding during the analysis of data. Two methods that readers will commonly encounter are control tables and multivariable analysis.

Control Tables

The control-table method is stratification ex post facto. Rather than arranging subjects by age groups, smoking habits, or blood pressure levels as the study design is being created, results are calculated within specified subdivisions.

An example of a confounding relationship that has perplexed researchers is the possible link between sugar consumption and heart disease. Back in the early 1960s, Yudkin and Roddy postulated that increased intake of sucrose might lead to coronary artery disease.[2] In a case-control study, they compared 20 subjects recovering from acute myocardial infarctions with 25 controls who were either healthy or were patients on an orthopedic ward. The mean sugar intake for the 2 groups differed considerably, as shown in Table 12–3. Heart disease patients reported consuming almost twice as much sugar as controls. These were provocative findings and stimulated other researchers to test the hypothesis.[3–5] In the course of this subsequent work, it became apparent that individuals who consumed large amounts of sugar had other habits that might be related to heart disease. They consumed substantial amounts of coffee and tea, and they smoked more. The relationship of smoking, which is a risk factor for heart disease, to sugar consumption has created a confounding problem. For purposes of illustration, let us use some hypothetical data to see how this confounding might work.

TABLE 12–3
Mean daily sugar consumption of 20 patients with heart disease and 25 control subjects

	Sugar consumption (g/day)
Heart disease patients (n = 20)	132
Control subjects (n = 25)	77

Modified, with permission, from Yudkin and Roddy.[2]

Yudkin's figures show that heart disease patients consume an average of 132 g of sugar per day, compared with 77 g daily for controls. If, however, people who eat more sugar also smoke more, and smokers are apportioned differently among cases and controls, the results might appear as in Table 12–4. The overall averages reflect the apparent association; but by evaluating sugar intake within subgroups of smoking and nonsmoking subjects, the effects of smoking are controlled. Once this is done, the relationship between sugar consumption and heart disease disappears. The mean sugar consumption for heart disease patients who smoke is almost identical to that of smoking control patients. Likewise, nonsmokers consume only 50 g of sucrose per day regardless of whether or not they have heart disease. Smoking is related to heart disease; sucrose intake is not. It is apparent, however, that for the relationship

TABLE 12–4
Mean daily sugar consumption of 20 patients with heart disease and 25 control subjects (controlled for smoking)

	Sugar consumption (g/day)
Heart disease patients (n = 20)	132
Smokers (n = 16)	152
Nonsmokers (n = 4)	50
Control subjects (n = 25)	77
Smokers (n = 7)	148
Nonsmokers (n = 18)	50

between sucrose and heart disease to completely disappear, smokers must be very unevenly distributed. Of the 20 heart attack patients, 16 must be smokers, compared with only 7 of the 25 controls, to achieve the results that were obtained.

Frequently, a confounding factor exerts an influence on results but is not entirely responsible for findings. When Elwood et al attempted to replicate Yudkin's work, they found that smoking indeed confounded the relationship between sugar consumption and heart disease, but that even when smoking was controlled, a small residual relationship remained.[5] Table 12–5 depicts two different ways our hypothetical data can be displayed. Both formats are encountered in medical articles and are referred to as *control tables*. Table 12–5(b) looks just like the two-by-two tables we used before to categorize subjects by diseases and characteristics, but it is a bit more complex. It shows the relationship between 3 rather than 2 variables. The figures in each box no longer represent the number of

---

TABLE 12–5
Relationship between mean daily sugar consumption and heart disease (with smoking as confounding factor)

	Sugar consumption (g/day)
(a)	
Heart disease patients ($n = 20$)	132
Smokers ($n = 12$)	152
Nonsmokers ($n = 8$)	101
Control subjects ($n = 25$)	77
Smokers ($n = 10$)	118
Nonsmokers ($n = 15$)	50

(b)

	Sugar consumption (g/day)	
	Heart disease	Controls
Smokers	152 ($n = 12$)	118 ($n = 10$)
Nonsmokers	101 ($n = 8$)	50 ($n = 15$)

subjects; they portray an attribute of the subjects—in this case, mean daily sugar consumption. Reading the rows of the control table, comparing smokers with nonsmokers, we find that regardless of whether subjects have heart disease or not, smokers have higher sugar consumption (152 g/day compared with 101 g/day, 118 g/day compared with 50 g/day). Inspecting the columns, we see that patients with heart disease also consume more sugar than patients without heart disease in both the smoking and the nonsmoking groups. The conclusion to be drawn from this table is that the relationship between sugar consumption and heart disease is in fact confounded by smoking. However, when the effect of smoking is held constant, the association between sucrose consumption and heart disease remains. Both smoking and sugar are related to heart problems.

The case-control study of Pap smear screening and prevention of cervical cancer (Chapter 6) recalls another example where confounding puts results at risk.[6] Investigators worried that because cases and controls were self-selected with respect to obtaining Pap smears, other risk factors might also be unequally distributed and be responsible for the cervical cancer. The mean age of the 2 groups was comparable, but socioeconomic status as measured by income and education was not. The average grade achieved in school was only 9.9 among cases compared with 11.1 for controls. Cases also had substantially lower family income on average. Social class, though mediated by other factors such as age at first intercourse, is a risk factor for cervical cancer. When the authors displayed their data (Table 12–6), they showed frequency of Pap smear screening stratified by age, income, and education. Relative risks of the same magnitude and direction are seen across the strata, and this indicates that confounding by these factors is not responsible for results.

Multivariable Analysis

Control tables are dandy for handling confounding variables when only one or two of the confusing factors are around. However, in many situations, several explanations are competing for causation credit. Human behavior is complex business. Heart disease has been linked to age, diet, personality type, blood pressure, cigarette smoking, and cholesterol level. Pregnancy outcome has been shown to be related to maternal age, race, socioeconomic status, parity, and marital status, to mention a few. Many of these causal factors are interrelated. When time comes to sort out just what is responsible for an outcome or effect, simple control tables are not

TABLE 12-6

Frequency of screening by Pap smear among cases and controls in relation to age, income, and education

	Frequency of Pap-smear screening		Relative risk
	Cases	Controls	
All subjects	67/212 (32%)	591/1060 (56%)	2.7
Age, years			
20-34	7/16 (44%)	66/107 (62%)	2.1
35-44	18/36 (50%)	124/185 (67%)	2.0
45-59	31/102 (30%)	266/460 (58%)	3.1
60+	11/58 (19%)	134/304 (44%)	3.4
Total	67/212 (32%)	590/1056 (56%)	2.8
Income ($)			
<6000	9/45 (20%)	81/184 (44%)	3.1
6-9999	9/41 (22%)	65/124 (52%)	3.9
10-14,999	12/37 (32%)	128/217 (59%)	3.0
15,000+	16/35 (46%)	160/226 (71%)	2.9
Total	46/158 (29%)	434/751 (58%)	3.2
Highest grade achieved			
<9	22/78 (28%)	109/251 (43%)	2.0
9-11	19/64 (30%)	200/339 (59%)	3.4
12+	19/43 (44%)	214/328 (65%)	2.4
Total	60/185 (32%)	523/918 (57%)	2.5

Modified, with permission, from Clarke and Anderson.[6]

up to the task. By the time we have tried to compare the sugar consumption of subjects who are of the same sex and age, smoke the same amount, have similar cholesterol levels, and have the same range of blood pressure, life has become exceedingly complex. The more factors we control in a data analysis, the smaller the number of subjects becomes in each subdivision and the larger samples must be to avoid incorrect inferences.

The multivariable regression models discussed in Chapter 9 are useful in this situation. In the Nurses Health Study report on the relationship between physical activity and coronary events, the risk of adverse coronary events decreased for every quintile of increasing physical activity (see Table 12–7).[7] We concluded that physical activity protects women against heart disease, but this result is loaded with opportunities for confounding. The most obvious one is age. As women grow older, they have

TABLE 12-7

Distribution of indicators of coronary risk and outcomes according to quintile group for total physical-activity score at baseline and relative risk of coronary events

Variable	Quintile group for total physical activity[a]				
	1	2	3	4	5
No. of women	13,859	15,065	14,598	14,326	14,640
Total physical activity score (MET-hour/week)					
Median	0.8	3.2	7.7	15.4	35.4
	Percentage of group				
Risk indicator					
Currently smoking	28.2	23.7	19.6	17.4	17.5
History of hypertension	26.1	25.1	24.0	22.4	21.0
History of diabetes	4.2	3.3	3.7	2.8	2.6
History of hypercholesterolemia	12.0	11.4	11.7	11.6	10.6
Current postmenopausal hormone replacement therapy	19.5	21.5	23.1	23.8	24.1
Use of multivitamin supplement	36.9	39.9	43.0	45.0	47.2
	Mean				
Age, years	52.1	52.3	52.2	52.2	52.3
Alcohol consumption (g/day)	5.9	5.8	6.0	6.4	7.0
Body mass index	25.1	24.6	24.2	23.9	23.5
	Outcomes				
No. of coronary events	178	153	124	101	89
Person-year of follow-up	106,252	116,175	112,703	110,886	113,419
	Relative risk				
Type of analysis					
Age-adjusted	1.0	0.77	0.65	0.54	0.46
Multivariate[b]	1.0	0.88	0.81	0.74	0.66

[a]The total physical activity score was expressed as MET-hours per week, calculated as the average time per week spent in each of 8 activities; multiplied by the MET value of each activity. The MET value is the caloric needs during exercise divided by the caloric needs at rest.
[b]The model included variables for age (in 5-year categories), period during the study (four 2-year periods), smoking status (never smoked, previously smoked, or currently smokes 1-14, 15-24, or ≥25 cigarettes per day), body mass index (in 5 categories), menopausal status (premenopausal, postmenopausal without hormone replacement therapy, postmenopausal with previous hormone replacement therapy, or postmenopausal with current hormone replacement therapy), parental history with respect to myocardial infarction before the age of 60 years, multivitamin supplement use, vitamin E supplement use, alcohol consumption (0, 1-4, 5-14, or ≥15 g/day), history of hypertension, history of diabetes, history of hypercholesterolemia, and aspirin use (none, 1-6 doses per week, or 7 or more doses per week).
Modified, with permission, from Manson et al.[7]

higher rates of heart disease. They also generally grow less active. Thus, the explanation for the relationship between heart disease and activity could be due to the confounding effects of age. Age is such a ubiquitous confounder that most investigators control for its potential mischief routinely in their analyses. The investigators for the Nurses Health Study did this, and the relative risks they present across the quintiles of activity in the first row of their analysis in Table 12–7 represent age-adjusted results.

However, there are other factors that could confound the relationship between physical activity and heart disease. Women who get more exercise are likely to differ from those who do not in other health-related ways. Examination of the table shows this is true for the nurse subjects. Nurses who have high physical activity smoke less and have less hypertension, diabetes, and high cholesterol than their less active colleagues. They are also more likely to use hormone replacement therapy (HRT) and multivitamins. Any of these factors might independently relate to the development of heart disease and thus act as a confounder. So the investigators throw a host of risk factors, such as these, into a multivariable model to create an estimate of relative risk that adjusts or controls for differences in risk factors across quintiles of physical activity. It is like using a control table except that the statistical model can adjust for all these variables at the same time.

The bottom row of Table 12–7 shows the relative risks obtained from the multivariable adjustments. These differ systematically from the estimates that were only age adjusted. Within each quintile of physical activity, the protective effect of activity has been mitigated. In the second quintile, it has gone from 0.77 to 0.88; in the fifth quintile, the relative risk is no longer 46% of that for the least active group, but 66%. This is as expected. Other risk factors, such as smoking and hypertension, are likely to contribute to coronary events. When they are taken into account, the impact of physical activity is diminished. However, its benefit persists. The relative risk for each of the quintiles of activity remains less than 1. To control for confounding, one must be able to identify, measure, and analyze the alternative explanations of study outcomes. These can be elusive and are not always easy to capture.

For some years, researchers from Brazil have been interested in the relationship between use of infant pacifiers and breast-feeding. Pacifiers, it turns out, are reputed to be culprits in the early termination of breast-feeding—a particular problem in developing countries where breast-feeding protects infants from a variety of infectious diseases. In one of several studies they conducted, 600 mothers were recruited at a maternity hospital for a 6-month follow-up study of infant feeding practices.[8] Mothers were interviewed at home visits conducted when their infants were 1, 4, and 6 months of age and queried about their infant feeding practices and use of pacifiers.

Results confirmed the investigators' fears. Over the course of 6 months, they found that as pacifier use increased, breast-feeding declined. Among infants for whom pacifier use was frequent at 1 month of age, only 20% were exclusively or predominantly breast-feeding by 4 months of age. This compared with a breast-feeding frequency of 57% for infants with no pacifier use at 1 month of age. The relative risk for weaning from the breast and using pacifiers was 3.8 (95% confidence interval, 2.7–5.5; $P < .001$). The authors realized, however, that other factors may contribute to stopping breast-feeding. These could confound the picture. They reckoned that socioeconomic status, demographic variables, parity, and other prenatal and infant feeding characteristics needed to be considered. Therefore, they used statistical modeling to adjust for these factors. Indeed, the relative risk dropped, indicating some confounding was occurring. But at 2.9, it was still statistically significant. The authors note that their study still does not guarantee a causal link between pacifier use and early weaning. Other unmeasured factors, such as poor infant sucking, might still confound their findings. They do, however, recommend that pacifiers not be used for breast-fed infants and that "mothers and families, particularly in developing countries, should be made aware of these facts and advise against the early introduction of pacifiers."[8]

A group of investigators from Montreal was not convinced. They organized a randomized controlled trial to assess the pros and cons of pacifiers.[9] A total of 258 mother-infant pairs were randomly assigned to 1 of 2 breast-feeding education programs. The key difference in the 2 approaches was the admonition to avoid pacifiers in the "experimental" condition. Baseline comparison of experimental and control groups showed them to be similar with respect to maternal age, education, infant birth weight, and a variety of factors, such as prior pregnancies, all of which might be related to successful breast-feeding outcomes. The intervention had an effect. Pacifier use was decreased in the experimental group; almost 39% of mothers in the experimental group avoided pacifier use altogether compared with only 16% of control subjects. However, this had no effect on duration of breast-feeding; 18.9% of mothers in the experimental group had weaned their infants prior to 3 months of age compared with 18.3% of those in the control group (relative risk, 1.0; 95% confidence interval, 0.6–1.7). Because investigators had noted small differences between groups in the percentage of mothers who were married and those who smoked during pregnancy, they carried out a logistic regression analysis to control for these differences. Findings were unchanged. Pacifier use had little effect on duration of breast-feeding.

As an added touch, the Montreal researchers analyzed their data as if they had done an observational study. This meant calculating the relative risk of weaning for infants who had been exposed to pacifiers and those who had not irrespective of their random assignment. Of babies who had ever been given pacifiers, 21% were weaned before the age of 3 months compared with only 11% of babies never given pacifiers (relative risk, 1.9). The authors conclude that pacifier use appears to be an unmeasured marker of other breast-feeding difficulties, such as reduced motivation to breast-feed, rather than a cause of early termination by itself. Despite the use of sophisticated multivariable modeling to control confounding, some undetected factors were at play in the observational studies.

MAKING ASSOCIATIONS INTO CAUSES

Tracking causes more often takes us through a labyrinth of streets than down a straight path. When we have stripped away bias, chance, and confounders and convinced ourselves that an exposure factor or intervention is directly and independently linked to a disease or outcome, we still may not have a complete picture. Even if we are convinced that Reye syndrome is directly related to aspirin ingestion, what is the exact cause of the illness? Does the drug act as a direct liver toxin? Why do only a handful of children who take aspirin contract the disease? Is the illness a response to a mix of factors including host susceptibility, concurrent viral illness, and the drug? The causes of even seemingly straightforward infectious diseases are surprisingly complex. It is overly simple, for example, to say that tuberculosis is caused by the tubercle bacillus. Although the infecting organism must be present for tuberculosis to occur, only 10–15% of individuals who are infected with the germ ever develop active tuberculosis. The bacillus is a necessary but not a sufficient cause for the illness. Host resistance, nutritional status, social isolation, and adaptability to stress also play a role. Discussions of cause can rapidly become metaphysical as well as biological.

There are several practical hints that readers can use to help decide whether the associations they read about are causal. Hill has published a classic essay on causation.[10] He describes 9 features of relationships that are useful in constructing a case for causation. These are (1) strength of the association, (2) consistency of the observed evidence, (3) specificity of the relationship, (4) temporality of the relationship, (5) biological gradient or dose-response, (6) biological plausibility, (7) coherence of the evidence, (8) experimental confirmation, and (9) reasoning by analogy. Much has been written about these criteria and, unfortunately, more dogma has developed that these are rules of evidence that must be satisfied than Hill intended.[11] Some of the ideas, such as the specificity of a relationship that requires that single causes lead to single effects, have not held up. Cigarette smoking and its apparent causal relationship to multiple adverse health outcomes is an example that comes to mind at once. Nevertheless, several of Hill's ideas continue to guide thinking about causality.

Strength of the Association

One bit of evidence that tips the association balance toward causality is the strength of the association. When the relative risk or relative odds are high, the argument for cause gains support. The overemployed but potent example used to illustrate the point is the association between cigarette smoking and lung cancer. Here, odds ratios (ORs) as high as 30 to 1 have been found. The statement that a heavy cigarette user is 30 times more likely to contract lung cancer than a nonsmoker is difficult to ignore. On the other hand, the case for causation is weakened when the magnitude of risk is low.

Relative risks as high as those found in studies that link cigarette smoking and lung cancer are not common. Many of the studies readers are likely to encounter have risk or ORs between 1 and 2. Several of the examples we have been exploring, such as Pap smears and cervical cancer, have been in $2\frac{1}{2}$ to $3\frac{1}{2}$ range. The risks surrounding adverse outcomes for postmenopausal HRT have varied widely according to the outcomes assessed. Relative risks for endometrial cancer caused by HRT have been large, in the neighborhood of eight- to tenfold. At present there is little debate that unopposed estrogen use in postmenopausal women is a "cause" of endometrial cancer. The relationship between HRT and breast cancer, on the other hand, has been more controversial. Here, relative risk estimates have ranged from 1.1 to 1.4. There is concern that "weak" associations such as this one may be more likely to be caused by bias than our eight- to tenfold increases in risk. That may be true. But we should be careful to remember that lower relative risk numbers may still indicate causal relationships. They may simply represent less dominant precipitating agents.

Nor should the unusually elevated risk ratio create credulity. Recall the case-control study that explored the relationship between phenylpropanolamine (PPA) used in over-the-counter cold medicines and appetite suppressants and hemorrhagic stroke.[12] The OR reported for PPA exposure from appetite suppressants and stroke among women was 16.58. That means that women with stroke were 17 times more likely to have ingested PPA than were controls—an impressive multiple. However, a close look at the data on which this estimate is based reveal that among 383 cases 6 took PPA in its weight loss formulation compared with only 1 of 750 controls. Although this difference was shown to be unlikely the result of chance (the P value was .02), the 95% confidence interval is very wide—compatible with risk ratios as large as 182 or as little as 1.5. Misclassification of exposure status among only a few cases or controls could have a substantial impact on this estimate of risk magnitude. We must still be comfortable that basic concerns for chance, bias, and confounding are satisfied before declaring cause.

Dose-Response Relationship

Anytime a risk factor comes in doses or gradients of exposure, it is reasonable to expect that the risk of disease should increase with higher levels of exposure. Again, cigarette smoking and lung cancer provide the perfect example, as the work of Doll and Hill[13] shows (see Figure 12–2). The more cigarettes people smoke, the more death rates go up, and that implies causality.

This same type of evidence has been used to strengthen the link between HRT and endometrial cancer. Weiss et al have shown that the risk of cancer is greater in women who have taken high-estrogen-content medication than for those who have consumed a lesser amount.[14] Table 12–8 demonstrates the rise in relative risk associated with increasing daily dosage.

The physical activity and heart disease example we have been exploring also shows a dose-response effect.[7] In this study, however, increasing exposure (more activity) decreases risk (see Table 12–7). The pattern of declining risk across the increasing quintiles of physical activity is a perfect example of a dose-response relationship. It boosts our confidence that the benefits of exercise are real.

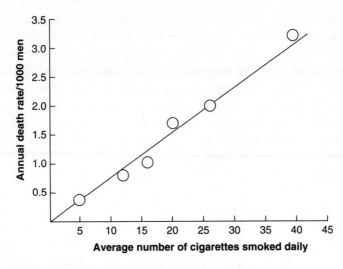

FIGURE 12-2. Annual death rate per 1000 men by average number of cigarettes smoked daily. (Modified, with permission, from Doll and Hill.[13])

On the other hand, the lack of a biological gradient where one might be expected should give pause for thought. To address a controversy over whether handheld cellular telephones are a risk factor for brain cancer, a group of investigators based in New York conducted a case-control study in five U.S. medical center hospitals.[15] The concern

	% of subjects			
Average dosage (mg/day)	**Endometrial cancer (n = 309)**	**Control (n = 272)**	**Relative risk**	**95% confidence interval**
Never used	20	63	1.0	...
≤0.5	5	7	2.5	1.1–5.3
0.6–1.2	32	12	8.8	5.0–12.7
≥1.25	44	18	7.6	5.0–11.6

TABLE 12-8

Menopausal estrogen use in women with endometrial cancer and controls according to average daily dosage

Modified, with permission, from Weiss et al.[14]

driving their investigation was that radio frequency signals emitted from handheld cell phones placed in close proximity to the head of the user might promote neoplastic changes in the brain.

The researchers identified 469 subjects with brain cancer. Controls were sought from the same hospital as each case and were matched by age, sex, race, and month of admission; 422 control subjects were found. Cases and controls were interviewed to determine their experience with cellular phones. It turned out that 14% of brain cancer patients reported using cellular telephones compared with 18% of control subjects. No increased risk here. However, reckoning that if any relationship between radio frequency exposure and brain cancer was to be found it should be more likely with increasing exposure, the researchers examined 3 potential dose-response relationships (Table 12–9). If cell phone use were related to cancer, increasing years of use, higher hours per month, and number of cumulative hours should provide a gradient that would uncover increasing risk. As the table illustrates, however, no such pattern appears for any of the three estimates—cooling any expectation that a causal relationship might be lurking in these data.

Biological Plausibility

To make a convincing argument for causation, the associations developed in medical studies should make biological sense. This means they should be consistent with information available from the related worlds of physiology, pharmacology, and anatomy. One argument that strengthens the case for estrogens as a cause for endometrial cancer has been the demonstration of concordance between the duration of exposure and development of disease. What we know of neoplasia suggests that cancers are not triggered immediately on exposure to a carcinogen, but instead develop after a latent period. We would expect that women exposed to estrogens would contract the neoplasm only some years after initial exposure. Table 12–10 depicts the increasing relative risk associated with the length of time since women were first exposed to estrogens. Women taking the medication for less than 3 years have essentially no increased risk of cancer.

The authors of the cell phone–brain cancer study also sought evidence of biological plausibility to support a link between brain cancer and cell phone use in their data. They reasoned that if radio frequency waves were responsible for inducing or promoting cancers, effects would be greatest closest to the source. They computed ORs in relation to the

TABLE 12–9
Odds ratios for brain cancer by amount and duration of handheld cellular telephone use

Cellular telephone use	No. (%) of cases (n = 469)	No. (%) of controls (n = 422)	Multivariable odds ratio (95% confidence interval)[a]	P for trend
No. of years				
0	403 (85.9)	346 (82.0)	1.0	.54
1[b]	21 (4.5)	30 (7.1)	0.7 (0.4–1.3)	
2–3	28 (6.0)	24 (5.7)	1.1 (0.6–2.0)	
≥4	17 (3.6)	22 (5.2)	0.7 (0.4–1.4)	
No. of hours/month				
0	403 (86.7)	346 (82.2)	1.0	.27
>0–≤0.72	19 (4.1)	20 (4.8)	1.0 (0.5–2.0)	
>0.72–≤2.1	10 (2.2)	17 (4.0)	0.5 (0.2–1.2)	
>2.1–≤10.1	20 (4.3)	18 (4.3)	0.9 (0.5–1.9)	
>10.1	13 (2.8)	20 (4.8)	0.7 (0.3–1.4)	
No. of cumulative hours[c]				
0	403 (86.7)	346 (82.2)	1.0	.30
>0–≤8.7	17 (3.7)	18 (4.3)	1.0 (0.5–2.0)	
>8.7–≤60	12 (2.6)	19 (4.5)	0.6 (0.3–1.3)	
>60–≤480	19 (4.1)	19 (4.5)	0.9 (0.5–1.8)	
>480	14 (3.0)	19 (4.5)	0.7 (0.3–1.4)	

[a]Adjusted for age, years of education, sex, race, study center, proxy subject, and month and year of interview.
[b]Four cases used a cellular telephone for half a year.
[c]Four cases and 1 control had missing data on frequency of use.
Modified, with permission, from Muscat et al.[15]

TABLE 12–10

**Menopausal estrogen use in women with endometrial cancer
and controls according to time since first use**

| Time since first use, years | % of subjects | | Relative risk | 95% confidence interval |
	Endometrial cancer ($n = 281$)	Control ($n = 251$)		
Never used	22	68	1.0	.:.
1–2	2	4	1.2	0.4–3.7
3–4	7	4	5.4	2.5–11.5
5–7	14	9	4.7	2.6–8.4
8–10	19	6	11.7	6.2–21.8
11–14	20	3	24.2	11.8–49.4
15–19	13	4	10.2	5.3–20.0
≥20	4	1	8.3	2.8–24.5

Modified, with permission, from Weiss et al.[14]

anatomical site of the tumors. No ORs significantly greater than 1 were observed by site, including the temporal lobe, the site closest to the exposure source. Again, there is little to support a causal relationship between cell phones and brain cancer.

Studies of the relationship between HRT and breast cancer have brought evidence of biological plausibility to bear in suggesting the causality of this relationship. When researchers have looked at age at menopause in relation to incidence of breast cancer among women who have never used HRT, for example, they have found that at a given age, premenopausal women have a higher relative risk of breast cancer than those who have gone through menopause.[16] This is true regardless of whether menopause is natural or surgically induced, and suggests that risk increases with the length of time of estrogen exposure. In a sense, HRT simply extends the duration of estrogen exposure beyond menopause. It has also been noted that increased risks of breast cancer associated with HRT are most pronounced for women with lower body mass index. This finding makes sense given the estrogen-producing capacity of adipose tissue in the body. Since postmenopausal women of lower weight should have lower levels of naturally occurring estrogens than their heavier contemporaries, the increase in hormones provided by HRT provides a bigger contrast and a bigger increase in relative risk.

Consistency of the Observed Evidence

Evidence ought to hang together in a consistent manner, both within the confines of a study and from one study to another. Once more, the HRT–breast cancer story provides an example. In the large collaborative effort that analyzed data from 51 epidemiologic studies,[16] investigators found a consistent pattern of small, increased relative risk of breast cancer for women ever-using HRT versus women never-using HRT. Although the point estimates of relative risk varied somewhat, they were generally above 1.0 and rarely exceeded 1.5. This was true for follow-up studies, case-control studies that used population controls, and case-control studies with hospital controls. When data are assessed for current or recent HRT users who have received treatment for 5 years or more, the same magnitude of relative risk across ethnic groups, education levels, parity, and a variety of other demographic characteristics is found. The risk numbers are consistently in the range of 1.2–1.5.

If an association between a factor and a disease is demonstrated time and time again through several studies that utilize different populations and different study techniques, the argument for causation is improved. On the other hand a lack of consistency in risk estimates should raise causal concerns. This can occur even within a single study. In the investigation of PPA and stroke,[12] the remarkably elevated OR of 17 was found for only 1 of 4 subsets of subject use, women, and appetite suppressants. The risk estimate for women exposed to PPA in cough or cold remedies was only 1.5 with a *P* value of .23 and 95% confidence interval that included 1. For male subjects neither use of PPA-containing cough/cold medications nor appetite suppressants was significantly associated with hemorrhagic stroke. We need explanations why differences in formulation or subject sex should alter risk.

SUMMARY

The search for causation always takes place under the ominous shadow of confounding. Characteristics that seem directly related to outcomes or diseases may be incorrectly identified as causal because of linkages with intermediary, confounding variables. Careful readers should ask these questions:

1. Have the authors addressed the possibility that chance, bias, or confounding factors are responsible for the effects they have observed?

2. Are the potential confounders identified? Is the list reasonable? Are any known risks not included? Could unmeasured confounders be playing a role?

3. Have steps been taken to control confounding? Was matching employed when the study design was created, or have multivariable techniques or control tables been employed in the analysis?

4. If authors have supplied evidence that potentially causal factors are not confounded, what additional evidence is there to suggest causality? Does evidence of the strength of the association, the biological plausibility, the consistency, and the dose-response relationship make a convincing case?

REFERENCES

1. Friedmann E et al: Animal companions and one-year survival of patients after discharge from a coronary care unit. Public Health Rep 1980;95:307.
2. Yudkin J, Roddy J: Levels of dietary sucrose in patients with occlusive atherosclerotic disease. Lancet 1964;2:6.
3. Bennett AE, Doll R, Howell RW: Sugar consumption and cigarette smoking. Lancet 1970;1:1011.
4. Burns-Cox CJ, Doll R, Ball KP: Sugar intake and myocardial infarction. Br Heart J 1969;31:485.
5. Elwood PC et al: Sucrose consumption and ischemic heart disease in the community. Lancet 1970;1:1014.
6. Clarke EA, Anderson TW: Does screening by "Pap" smears help prevent cervical cancer? A case-control study. Lancet 1979;2(8132):1.
7. Manson JE et al: A prospective study of walking as compared with vigorous exercise in the prevention of coronary heart disease in women. N Engl J Med 1999;341(9):650.
8. Barros FC et al: Use of pacifiers is associated with decreased breast-feeding duration. Pediatrics 1995;95(4):497.
9. Kramer MS et al: Pacifier use, early weaning, and cry/fuss behavior: A randomized controlled trial. JAMA 2001;286(3):322.

10. Hill AB: The environment and disease: Association or causation? Proc R Soc Med 1965;58:295.

11. Rothman K, Greenland S: *Modern Epidemiology,* 2nd ed. Lippincott-Raven, 1998.

12. Kernan WN et al: Phenylpropanolamine and the risk of hemorrhagic stroke. N Engl J Med 2000;343:1826.

13. Doll R, Hill AB: Mortality in relation to smoking: Ten years' observations of British doctors. Br Med J 1964;1:1399.

14. Weiss NS et al: Endometrial cancer in relation to patterns of menopausal estrogen use. JAMA 1979;242:261.

15. Muscat JE et al: Handheld cellular telephone use and risk of brain cancer. JAMA 2000;284(23):3001.

16. Collaborative Group on Hormonal Factors in Breast Cancer. Breast cancer and hormone replacement therapy: Collaborative reanalysis of data from 51 epidemiological studies of 52,705 women with breast cancer and 108,411 women without breast cancer. Lancet 1997;350(9084):1047.

CHAPTER THIRTEEN

Case Series Editorials, and Reviews

*We are constantly misled by the ease with which our minds
fall into the ruts of one or two experiences.*

SIR WILLIAM OSLER

W e have devoted a good bit of energy to critical evaluation of research studies that look for explanations or evaluate therapies. In doing so, we have neglected the large numbers of studies that we classified as descriptive back in Chapter 2. By "descriptive," we refer to papers in which authors review their experience managing patients at the end of life, or where they catalog the depressed patients who present to their family practice clinic. The goal of these papers is not to explore hypotheses about cause or to test a new treatment but to share experience that may be useful to readers. The prototype of these descriptions is the case report or case series, in which groups of patients are classified and summarized according to their blood pressure, activities of daily living changes, length of hospital stay, or any of a multitude of features of interest. We noted earlier that a case series may be the first step toward more sophisticated research.

CASE SERIES

Adverse Events

Sometimes a series of cases is all that is needed to shatter a shibboleth or demonstrate exceptions to a rule. Case reports can announce the occurrence of previously unsuspected adverse drug effects or show that joggers are not immune from heart attacks. Timeliness is usually a feature of this use of the case series. The information provided is often preliminary and methodologically unrefined, but it has a legitimate place in journal pages because it is "newsworthy."

In the midst of great public concern over the "epidemic" use of cocaine in the United States, Isner et al[1] worried that there was a misperception that the drug is "not associated with serious medical complications." The authors describe 7 cases of young adults who experienced ventricular fibrillation, myocarditis, and myocardial infarction associated with cocaine use. Their message is simple: "Recreational cocaine use may be very dangerous." The authors caution against interpreting the associations as establishing a clean, causal relationship between cocaine and cardiovascular disorders. They admit that their evidence is circumstantial. Without a denominator, we have no idea what proportion of all cocaine users these 7 cases represent. Without comparisons, we cannot be certain that the number of cardiac events Isner et al described is not simply the expected rate in the overall population of young adults, regardless of their exposure to cocaine. Interpretation must proceed with caution. Still, the readership becomes more attentive to the drug's possible cardiotoxicity.

In our striving for perfection of size, shape, and performance, Americans have come to consume large amounts of dietary supplements. Some of these may do more harm than good. Ma huang, a supplement containing ephedra alkaloids, which is promoted for weight reduction and energy enhancement, is a case in point. Investigators from the University of California performed an in-depth review of 140 reports submitted to the U.S. Food and Drug Administration that claimed possible adverse reactions to ephedra-containing supplements.[2] The challenge of the project was to properly attribute causality to the ephedra using case reports only— without the benefits of a control group. The researchers constructed a classification scheme utilizing causation criteria such as those we discussed in the last chapter. For example, the timing of events needed to be consistent with when the drug was administered, and the nature of events needed to fit with recognized side effects of ephedrine (the active compound). Subjects' concurrent medical conditions and other, potentially confounding exposures were also considered in the review.

Forty-three subjects were rated as definitely or probably related and 44 others were put in the possible category. Most adverse events involved the cardiovascular or central nervous system, including a number of fatalities. These serious outcomes are known to be associated with the drug. However, could confounding be occurring here? Could subjects have predisposing medical conditions or be taking other potentially toxic drugs? Absolutely. Some of the reported products also contain caffeine and other known stimulants. But even if the case reports are not conclusive, they do raise our level of suspicion. We are put on notice, and, given the lack of evidence that the supplements produce the weight loss or increased energy that is claimed, avoiding Ma huang seems prudent.

Cataloging the New

Sometimes a novel disease or an outbreak of an illness is uncommon or new to a particular locale. As the world shrinks, health problems have become global. Diseases caused by West Nile virus make appearances on the East Coast of the United States. Antibiotic-resistant salmonella cross the Pacific Ocean from the Philippines and cause outbreaks of disease in Oregon nursing homes. Travelers return from exotic lands with some unwanted souvenirs. Descriptive accounts of these experiences, their clinical presentations, and demographic features can be helpful.

Suppose you are a clinician responsible for the well-being of students and faculty at a large university in the northeastern United States. Into the clinic strolls a middle-aged professor with complaints of fever for a week, an unpleasant skin ulcer on his leg, and a vesicular rash of the trunk and forearms. By the way, he reports having just returned from South Africa 2 weeks ago, where he had been wandering on the veldt. As you puzzle over this presentation, it occurs to you that several weeks ago you scanned an article in the *New England Journal of Medicine* that had to do with a tick-transmitted disease found in sub-Saharan Africa. You retreat to the stack of journals on your desk (or the Web site for the journal) and locate the article on African tick-bite fever.[3] The study reports on 119 cases of *Rickettsia africae* infection, most of which occurred in South Africa. You locate a table of signs and symptoms associated with the illness and note that your patient's characteristics fit beautifully with those described. You also note that 74% of the patients in the series were treated with doxycycline and recovered uneventfully. While there are no guarantees that similarities with the study findings assure us our patient has African tick-bite fever or that doxycycline would be the treatment of choice were it subjected to a randomized trial, we know more than we did before.

Health Services Planning

Let us suppose that we have been appointed to a committee to plan a new hospital geriatrics unit. In the course of meetings, questions arise concerning staffing needs and service requirements for the new unit. What will be the anticipated length of stay for a typical patient? What disabilities will patients have, and how frequently will these occur? Will patients need help with their daily activities? Will impaired mental status be a problem, necessitating special supervision? A study published by Warshaw et al provides guidelines to answer some of these questions.[4] Though technically this study employs a prevalence or cross-sectional design that relates increasing age to increasing functional disability, much of its value lies in documenting the types and extent of functional impairment among hospitalized elderly. The paper reports on a survey conducted in a 400-bed community hospital. Over 250 patients aged 70 years or above were assessed on functional variables such as mental status, impaired hearing and vision, and ability to perform activities of daily living. Demographic information and features of the hospitalization such as length of stay and services required were also documented. Selected results are shown in Table 13–1.

TABLE 13–1
Functional impairment among 279 hospitalized elderly patients

| | | | Needing assistance | | Impaired | |
Confused	Incontinent	Confined to chair or bed	Eating	Dressing	Vision	Hearing
50%	21%	33%	38%	53%	40%	34%

Modified, with permission, from Warshaw et al.[4]

These findings could be useful to our committee. Warshaw et al found that the average elderly patient stayed in the hospital 21 days, with a range from 2 to 126 days. Of these patients, 34 and 40% had hearing and vision impairment, respectively. Many needed help with eating or dressing, including over 50% of the 39 patients who were 85 years of age or older. Fifty percent of patients had exhibited some degree of mental confusion, a problem that was also more prevalent among the oldest patients. We need to plan accordingly.

The personal experience of any one of us is limited, no matter how many our years. Reports of series of cases enlarge our experience with only a few flips of the page. Moreover, our recollections of the details of the cases we have seen dim with time. Often they are selected by the dramatic episode rather than guided by the usual instance. We are more likely to recall the one or two cases of Stevens-Johnson syndrome that occurred after sulfonamide was given for a urinary tract infection rather than the 100 uneventful courses of the drug. We might remember the hospital experiences of some of our elderly patients, but we are unlikely to recall that the average length of stay in this population reaches 3 weeks or that as many as 50% of these patients have some degree of confusion. The case series broadens our view and sharpens our faulty memories.

At the same time, we must remember important critical concerns such as external validity. Do patients from the medical center behave like those I care for? Is there any reason to believe that their cases of meningitis are any more or less severe or respond to treatment differently from those in patients I treat? Are the elderly admitted to the community hospital where Warshaw et al worked typical of my setting? Do my patients tend to be as old, stay as long, or have the same proportion of orthopedic and urological problems? We must have some indication that these study populations are similar to our own before we can feel comfortable embracing the findings of these descriptive studies.

Therapy

We have stated that one feature of the case series is that it does not pretend to evaluate treatments. That rule is often broken. There are many reports of new operations, drug regimens, or health service improvements in which a series of patients is subjected to an intervention and our insistence on a proper control group is ignored. To be sure, there are instances in which treatment of a series of patients produces such dramatic results that even serious skeptics are won over and their cries of protest are temporarily silenced. The effects of insulin on diabetic hyperglycemia, of penicillin on pneumococcal pneumonia, or of vitamin B_{12} on pernicious anemia have been accepted without demands for randomized trials. However, these examples of "slam-bang effects," as Moses calls them, are not common.[5] Moreover, there is a grave risk that uncontrolled case-series studies will proclaim "slam-bangers" when they should not. Reports of internal mammary artery ligation for angina, gastric freezing for peptic ulcer disease, and diethylstilbestrol for threatened abortion all broke loudly on the scene. Now each is only a whispered embarrassment of the past.

Bailar et al include case-series studies in a discussion of "studies without internal controls."[6] They argue that studies that lack simultaneously-followed comparison subjects almost always have "implicit controls." These include historic controls, such as patients from the same clinic who had the older method of gallbladder surgery, or community controls, such as the percentage of patients in the county who had rubella in the year prior to the introduction of the new vaccine. Sometimes these "external controls" come from previously published reports on the same issue. Sometimes they are culled from "common knowledge," implying there is standard agreement; for example, that prior to the introduction of penicillin, all patients with subacute bacterial endocarditis died of the disease. We have discussed the frailties of the nonconcurrent, nonrandomized comparison subject enough so that these "implicit controls" must be viewed with skepticism. On the other hand, some useful information about new treatments can come from case-series studies.

A. Feasibility and Safety: A case series is a reasonable way to find out whether a new intervention is feasible. Is an innovative surgical procedure technically possible? Can patients tolerate a new cancer therapeutic agent? Can home health care be provided for terminally ill patients at a reasonable cost?

A group of cardiothoracic surgeons from Germany offer a descriptive study on a high-tech approach to cardiac surgery.[7] Two hundred and one patients underwent robotically assisted coronary artery bypass grafting. Immediate success rates were excellent, with a survival rate of 99%. Only 9 patients required reexploration. No assessment of randomized interventions here, just the first reports on the feasibility and potential efficacy of a new technique. Will robotically assisted surgery produce better results than conventional techniques? Will it be safer or more cost-effective?

Answers to such questions must be supplied by other investigators. This case series gives them a place to start.

Induction of abortion through the sequential administration of two orally administered pills, mifepristone and misoprostol, has been shown in European trials to be efficacious. However, the drugs are expensive and, as administered in Europe, require 3 or more clinic visits. This complexity and cost restrict the usefulness of the treatment in less developed countries. Researchers from the Population Council conducted a trial in two countries, Vietnam and Tunisia, using a much simplified regimen.[8] They reduced the dosage of the most expensive of the drugs to one-third and arranged for women to have only one clinic visit where they received mifepristone and were given the option of home administration of the second drug several days later. All subjects were treated. There was no random allocation, double-blinding, or placebos in evidence. Investigators focused on compliance with the protocol, efficacy of the drugs in achieving abortion, and side effects. They found that the treatment with the reduced dosage and home administration resulted in better than 90% compliance and 90% success. The frequency of unusually heavy bleeding was small, and no women required a blood transfusion. Pain and abdominal cramping lasted only a few days.

The study is reminiscent of the effectiveness trials we discussed in Chapter 6. Although randomized controlled trials of the drug combination had been performed earlier and demonstrated the success of the combination, this uncontrolled case series tested the feasibility of an important variation on the regimen. The reduced dosage of mifepristone produced successful results, and the home administration of misoprostol met with high compliance and patient satisfaction. This was a reasonable result despite the absence of a rigorous design.

B. Potential Efficacy: Randomized clinical trials are difficult to organize and are usually costly. Some indication of efficacy of a new intervention must be available before elaborate studies can be justified. The case series can serve this preliminary screening function.

Many anecdotes supporting the benefits of amygdalin (Laetrile) in the treatment of cancer spawned passionate debate among lay persons and health professionals over licensing and use of the drug.[9] Amygdalin is a natural, cyanide-containing derivative of apricot pits and has been used as an ingredient in herbal medications for centuries. The U.S. Food and Drug Administration refused to approve the use of Laetrile despite the testimonials of many cancer patients that they had experienced remarkable effects. Because opinions about Laetrile were so divided, the National Cancer Institute sponsored a large case-series study to see if any benefits of the compound could be demonstrated.

Investigators from 4 major medical centers across the United States collaborated to assess Laetrile's potential. Patients enrolled in the study had histologically proven cancer for which no standard, efficacious treatment was available. They were accepted only if they were ambulatory, able to maintain oral nutrition, and in generally good condition. To be eligible, each patient had to have a tumor that could be objectively measured. Laetrile therapy was guided by the practices described by proponents of the drug. Dosages and methods of administration were chosen to be representative of current practice, and adjuvant "metabolic therapy" diets, including high-dose vitamins and pancreatic enzymes, were added so as to parallel programs used by practitioners of Laetrile therapy. To assess results of treatment, objective criteria for response, stability, or progression of disease based on tumor size and metastatic involvement were defined. By selecting basically "healthy" cancer patients, using the full doses and adjuvant treatment recommended by Laetrile practitioners, and establishing objective guidelines to measure response, investigators intended to maximize the opportunity to detect benefits of the treatment.

The results were compelling. A total of 179 patients were entered into the study. By the completion of 3 weeks of intravenous amygdalin therapy, 54% of the 175 evaluable patients had measurable progression of their disease. Three months after initiation of therapy, 91% demonstrated disease progression; by 7 months, disease had progressed in all. Only 7% of patients with impaired performance status prior to therapy claimed any improvement during treatment, and only 20% claimed any symptomatic relief anytime during therapy. Survival data were no more promising. The median survival of all patients was less than 5 months from the start of treatment (Figure 13–1).

As Relman remarked in an accompanying editorial, "This study closes the books on Laetrile."[10] The research, born out of urgent public concern that the medical establishment was "withholding" valuable cancer therapy, was not controlled, not randomized, and not blind. All patients were given Laetrile, and both patients and investigators knew what drug was being administered. In a "triumph of pragmatism over principle, it [the study] got the job done."[10] The rapid progression of disease and limited survival of the cancer patients provided no evidence of beneficial effect. The case-series results precluded the need for randomized, controlled trials.

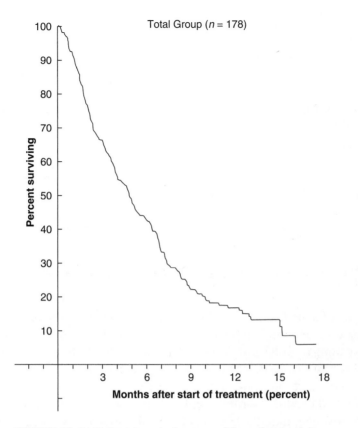

FIGURE 13–1. Patients' survival measured from the start of amygdalin treatment. (Reprinted, with permission, from Moertel et al.[9])

A twist on the uncontrolled study of efficacy theme is seen in research that looks for benefits not from starting but from stopping treatment. As suggested earlier, using patients as their "own controls" is chancy business. In some cases, however, it seems rather reasonable. Concerned that a proportion of patients receiving long-term antihypertensive treatment may no longer require medication prompted a study of treatment withdrawal in 18 participating general practices in the northeast of England.[11] Collaborating practices selected approximately 200 patients who had been treated with antihypertensive medication for some years. Patients were withdrawn from medication according to a standardized protocol and were followed up for 3 years. Patients returned for blood pressure monitoring every several months during this interval. By the end of the study 22% of the subjects remained normotensive without their medication. Of those who required reinstitution of treatment, most were restarted within 3 months. Although a concurrent control group and random allocation were not part of this experiment, it is difficult to imagine that their presence would have enhanced the internal validity of results. However, a usual caveat applies. The final study population was selected after 2805 possible hypertensive patients had been screened. Only 723 had optimal control and were without excluding conditions such as recent cardiovascular events or other reasons to require the medications. Of those, only 224 were successfully recruited and 196 followed up. It becomes difficult to determine just whom these final patients represent.

EDITORIALS & LETTERS TO THE EDITOR

A section of a medical journal that we have slighted is the editorial pages. Many journal editors highlight a paper they feel is particularly noteworthy by calling on colleagues to comment on the study. Often the commentary provides a context for the research by reviewing the current state of work in the area and reflecting on the significance of the new paper. Sometimes an editorial writer offers methodological critique as well. This can be most helpful to those of us who are trying to assess the merits of a study.

Two studies employed similar, case-control designs that utilized the same General Practice Research Database to test an observation that statin drugs prescribed to lower lipids might have the added benefit of reducing bone fractures. The studies reached different conclusions, however. The first, from a Swiss pharmacoepidemiology unit, matched 3900 patients with fractures and 23,000 controls, all taken from a large database of more than 3 million general practice patients from the United Kingdom.[12] When use of statin compounds among cases and controls was compared, a reduction in fracture risk of almost 50% was found for patients taking statins (adjusted odds ratio, 0.55; 95% confidence interval, 0.44–0.69). The second study, conducted by British and Dutch researchers, used the same general practice database to address the same question.[13] This study had 81,000 fracture cases and 81,000 matched controls. However, after adjusting the data for potential confounders, such as body mass index, smoking status, and other medications, these investigators came up with an odds ratio of 1.01 (95% confidence interval, 0.88–1.16). In the course of discussion, the investigators offered explanations for why their results (the correct findings in their view) differed from those in the earlier Swiss report.

Debate ensued in subsequent letters to the editor.[14] The Swiss team responded by identifying aspects of methodology in the British-Dutch report they viewed as unsatisfactory, such as failure to exclude certain patients at particularly high risk for fracture and techniques of matching. The British-Dutch group responded in turn. They defended their methods by presenting reanalyses of data that addressed criticisms. Revised odds ratios matched their original estimates. This all makes for stimulating reading. It also gives insight into methodological nuances that extends beyond the original published papers—an educational exercise.

The editorial pages also host debates on controversies of the day. A journal editor emeritus and pharmaceutical representative sparred over pharmaceutical industry support of continuing medical education. Dr. Relman argues that the pharmaceutical industry has "gone too far," decrying the fact that continuing medical education with its heavy financial support from drug companies is becoming a tool of pharmaceutical marketing rather than the provider of unbiased medical information.[15] He cites published evidence that industry-supported education activities are biased in favor of the sponsors' products and that the physicians who attend such courses prescribe the products more often than those of their competitors. Mr Holmer counters that "the accelerating pace of biomedical progress . . . makes it more imperative than ever for physicians to stay abreast of the latest medical innovations and treatments."[15] He lauds the pharmaceutical industry for playing "a leading role" in sponsoring the continuing education that will help physicians meet these needs.

Letters with New Data

Occasionally letters to the editor include brief summaries of the letter writer's own scientific observations.

A group of physicians from Verona, Italy, weighed in on the debate on fracture risk and statin use.[16] Noting the previously published articles under discussion were in disagreement, they contributed their own set of observations from a study they were conducting on osteoporosis among healthy men in their district. They obtained bone mineral density examinations as well as blood lipid levels on 427 healthy men. They then compared cholesterol levels with bone mineral density and found that subjects with the worst lipid profiles had the highest bone density values. Since statins are more likely to be prescribed to patients with high cholesterol levels, the association noted in studies suggesting statins *induced* higher bone mass might be an artifact of confounding. Another perspective is added to the debate.

Because letters are usually limited to brief reports and preliminary observations, they rarely include detailed methodology. Nor are letters sent out for peer review, as are more substantial works of original research. Relman has issued a caveat emptor concerning data contained in letters in an editorial entitled, "How reliable are letters?"[17] "There is a risk that uncritical readers may be misled if they fail to appreciate the tentative and incomplete nature of the evidence contained in these letters."

REVIEWS

Review articles are intended to bring us up-to-date on the risks of passive smoking, state of the art of prophylactic use of antibiotics in surgery, or of diagnosis and management of arthritis, and the like. Reviews can condense a great amount of material into a few pages. They save us the trouble of pacing the dusty stacks or pounding the keyboard to track down primary sources, and hours of reading and organizing data. Most reviews focus on content. Their aim is to present a large amount of information on a subject comprehensively and efficiently. Writers of reviews are often acknowledged as experts in their fields and frequently have conducted research themselves. However, it is not enough to have command of the literature on beta-blockers or thyroid function. Reviews have their own set of methodological pitfalls to trap the unwary. Writers and readers of reviews must bring along their critical appraisal skills. Reviews are particularly susceptible to biases in the selection and interpretation of the papers that comprise them.

Selection

Writers of reviews should note where they looked for primary sources and what selection criteria were used to include papers in the review.

Finding all the research reports on a topic is not easy. Resources such as computerized searches may include only a portion of published work. Pertinent studies may appear in journals that are not indexed or that are simply missed by indexers because keywords that are used to place papers into headings differ from those that the reviewers are using in their research. Sacks et al have noted that computer searches of the literature may yield less than two-thirds of relevant papers.[18] They suggest the use of *Current Contents,* other reviews, and experts in the field as additional resources.

Methodological Critique

The literature on any topic can be a methodological hodgepodge, running the gamut from opinionated case reports to sophisticated controlled trials. It is not enough for a review to summarize the findings of research studies; some comment should be made on the research design and methodological quality of the work. The results of an uncontrolled series of 7 patients given Bull Durham's Extract for fatigue cannot be given equal value with a carefully controlled trial comparing Bull Durham's with Lydia Pinkham's Compound.

In reviewing the effects of anabolic steroids on athletic performance, Haupt and Rovere summarize the results of more than 20 published studies.[19] The authors cover an extensive list of issues, including effects of steroids on body weight, cardiovascular performance, and strength. As part of their review, they categorize study results according to features of experimental design such as number of subjects, presence or absence of controls, and blinding.

Fourteen studies demonstrated that athletes taking anabolic steroids increased their strength; 10 showed no significant improvement. The authors note the methodological limitations of several of the studies. One uncontrolled study had only 3 subjects, all of whom were championship weight lifters who were, according to the original researchers, of such a level of expertise that a comparable control group was unavailable. Of the 14 studies demonstrating improved strength among athletes, the authors note that only 7 were properly blinded to avoid the possibility of placebo effect. Of the 10 studies that failed to show a strength increase, 9 employed a proper double-blind protocol. Haupt and Rovere go on to discuss the possible effect that these limitations of design, and particularly the placebo effect, may have on interpretation of results of this research. By combining their content review with methodological critique, they help the reader interpret the results of their review.

Meta-analysis/Pooling

One review technique readers should know about goes by the lofty title "meta-analysis." Meta-analyses critically review research studies and statistically combine their data to help answer questions that are beyond the power of single papers. And "power" is just the term to describe the value of this technique. Combining data from several studies increases the sample size. Larger samples mean more precise estimates of rates or risks, or—in the case of clinical trials—a lesser likelihood of a type II error. Combining data from several small clinical trials on the same subject may reveal a clinically important difference in treatments that the individual small trials lacked the power to detect.

   Although the effects of exercise on glycemic control in Type 2 diabetics have been assessed in several small clinical trials, the findings have varied and lacked clear direction. A group of Canadian researchers performed a meta-analysis in hopes of clarifying the situation.[20] As a first step, they conducted an extensive literature search using computerized databases, references from textbooks, and published articles. They searched under a variety of headings and keywords in an effort to identify all published articles involving human subjects who were subjected to clinical trials that evaluated exercise in Type 2 diabetes. The search yielded approximately 2700 possible studies to review. Investigators winnowed this list by eliminating those without control groups, a specified exercise training program, an intervention duration of at least 8 weeks, or several other criteria they identified as minimal expectations. The eligible trials plummeted to 14 controlled comparisons of subjects with diabetes who were placed on an exercise regimen and had glycemic control monitored. The trials were all small, ranging from 10 to 31 subjects in the intervention groups with a total of 251 subjects in all. Of the 14 trials, 11 were randomized controlled trials and 3 were nonrandomized trials. Glycemic control was measured by glycosylated hemoglobin, an indicator of longer-term diabetes control. Data were abstracted from each published report and a statistical analysis was performed that combined estimates of the effect of the intervention on glycemic control for each of the studies, while accounting for baseline differences in numbers of subjects, and baseline glycosylated hemoglobin levels among the studies.

Results indicated that there were no significant baseline differences in glycosylated hemoglobin between experimental and control groups. There was, however, in the combined estimate, a significant drop in glycosylated hemoglobin in the exercise group compared with controls. This indicated improved diabetic control due to the exercise and was a finding deemed to be both statistically and clinically significant. Such evidence of benefit from the exercise programs was not unanticipated. Estimates that favored treatment had come from 12 of the 14 published trials. However, largely because of the small sample sizes of each of these prior endeavors, only 2 of the 12 estimates had 95% confidence intervals that excluded 1 (no difference). The confidence interval surrounding the estimate of benefit from the meta-analysis, on the other hand, was much narrower and clearly indicated the benefits of exercise.

This is a potent technique. A disparate collection of small studies with indeterminant findings has been synthesized into a single summary with a solid conclusion. Meta-analyses have become popular, appearing frequently in a range of medical journals. As a means to summarize a complex and often confusing body of research, meta-analysis seems to offer an almost magical solution.

But not everyone agrees that meta-analysis is such a good idea. There are critics as well as potential problems. Much of the debate has centered on what advocates consider the beauty of the process, *heterogeneity.* Is it legitimate to combine data from different studies using different populations, with varying treatments, different doses, and different durations? Does it make sense to force all these flavors into a single stew? In the exercise and diabetes meta-analysis, for example, subjects came from 8 different countries, had different mean ages, took different concurrent medications, and did not even participate in the same kind of exercise program. Some folks cycled, some walked, some jogged, and some lifted weights. Advocates of meta-analysis consider heterogeneity of studies a good thing. If results hold up across populations and withstand variations in the interventions under scrutiny, it adds robustness and external validity to the results. Obviously, variables in studies need to share sufficient common ground to make combining results sensible. In the exercise-diabetes example, varying exercise activities were all translated into standard energy-intensity equivalence (the METS we discussed in Chapter 6).

Another concern relates to our old friend selection bias. This can manifest its ugly head several ways. The goal of meta-analysis is the comprehensive synthesis of research in a given area. To be comprehensive authors must identify all the research on a topic. Therefore, studies large or small, positive or negative should be included. But this is not always so easily accomplished. Computerized databases that catalog publications make the job easier. However, successful searching depends on proper indexing of keywords so that some sophistication and experience are required to use the resource successfully. There is evidence that different researchers with differing experience using the same database can come up with differing lists of studies.[21] Nor are all the relevant research endeavors reported in English. A truly comprehensive meta-analysis should consider those as well.

Research studies cannot be retrieved from any database in any language if they are not published. A major concern in the meta-analysis field has been whether published studies offer a true representation of all the work that has been conducted. Most agree this is not the case. There is a tendency for authors to submit and for journals to publish studies with positive findings. Again, there is evidence that this occurs.[21] *Publication bias* slants the results of a meta-analysis toward positive findings. (Of course, publication bias is operating in the literature regardless of whether or not a meta-analysis is conducted.)

It is incumbent on researchers who are selecting studies for inclusion in the meta-analysis to be unbiased. Criteria for selection of articles must be determined in advance and researchers, like investigators in clinical trials, must not be influenced in their choices by the results they hope to find. Quality controls must also be in place to check the accuracy of data abstraction. As with any measurement activity, errors, both random and biased, can occur.

And what of the quality of the papers that make up the meta-analysis? Syntheses composed of inferior ingredients are unlikely to turn out as savory dishes. Much discussion has centered on the quality of trials that are included in meta-analyses and how such determinations are made.[21] In an effort to address the problem, a variety of checklists and scoring systems have been devised to assess article quality.[22] We will examine these in Chapter 14.

It can become rather confusing. While in-depth discussions go beyond our present purposes, useful details are available.[21] For most readers, simply seeking evidence that authors are aware of potential limitations and have attempted to remedy these is the best course of action. It is an approach we have taken throughout our discussions. In the exercise-diabetes example the authors are rigorous in their pursuit of research on the topic. In addition to utilizing familiar medically oriented databases, they examine databases devoted to sports and registries of dissertation abstracts, as well as perform "hand searches" of published articles that were located. They even consult expert colleagues in the field to identify unpublished work. The meta-analysis specifically includes non-English studies.

The exercise-diabetes study authors also address problems of selection bias and quality in their analysis. At the outset they established clear criteria for data inclusion. When data from the original studies were lacking or unclear, primary authors were contacted for clarification. Two of the meta-analysts independently performed literature searches, quality assessment, and data extraction. Disagreements in their assessments were resolved by conferring with the third author. Methodological quality was assessed using a well-recognized, published scale. Publication bias was assessed by using one of several techniques available. Their thoroughness should give readers some confidence that the authors are aware of the ingredients essential to meta-analysis and have incorporated them appropriately into their analytic recipe.

Meta-analysis has also been used to combine results of risk-factor-seeking observational studies. This use of the technique prompts even greater concern over heterogeneity, considering the variety of approaches—from case-control to cohort studies—that are available in the literature. However, given the importance of many questions of risk, some prudent attempts to synthesize observational research findings seem warranted. An example is the relationship we have discussed between hormone replacement therapy and breast cancer. An ambitious data-combining activity was undertaken by the Collaborative Group on Hormonal Factors in Breast Cancer.[23] In an effort to gather consensus on this important question, data were sought from all observational studies that addressed the risk. Sixty-three were discovered. However, rather than performing the traditional meta-analysis, which utilizes *summary risk estimates* from each study, these investigators solicited *original data* from the primary researchers. Their objective was to reanalyze these combined data. The activity is referred to as *data pooling*.

Of the 63 eligible studies that were identified, 51 provided original data: 49 from published reports and 2 from unpublished work. Original data were not available from the remaining work. The 51 studies in the reanalysis represented 21 countries and both case-control and cohort methodologies. Ultimately, data on 52,000 women with invasive breast cancer and 108,000 controls without breast cancer were analyzed. As might be imagined, problems of heterogeneity were considerable. Investigators were confronted with challenges of standardizing diagnoses, types and dosages of hormone replacement, and timing and diagnosis of menopause. They converted data from cohort studies into nested case-control designs so that data could be handled in a uniform design frame.

Once the methodological challenges of creating uniform definitions and converting data to common formats were met, however, the power of the study to provide useful information was substantial. A clear pattern of risk for cancer emerged. Current and very recent users of hormone replacement therapy have a slight increase in risk for breast cancer for each year of use. Among the group of active users who receive hormone replacement therapy for 5 years or longer (the average was 11 years), the relative risk is 1.35 (95% CI, 1.21–1.49). With the relatively narrow confidence interval, the combined results provide a more precise estimate of the risk than we have had before. A useful synthesis has taken place.

SUMMARY

Case-series studies, editorials, and review articles are journal offerings that can add substance to our reading fare.

1. The case series can give a first glimpse of exciting new findings or demonstrate exceptions to the rule. These descriptive studies can provide data on the natural history of disease or offer experience to guide health services. The feasibility and potential effectiveness of new treatments can be evaluated. But all the interpretation risks of subject selection and absent controls attend. *Caveat emptor!*

2. Editorials and letters to the editor present thought-provoking alternative interpretations and methodological insights. They may also give testimony to the wit, good humor, and even poetic talent of our colleagues.

3. Reviews offer efficient reading, but readers should ask: (a) Have the authors performed a thorough literature review, or presented only selected research findings? (b) Have they accepted the primary researchers' interpretation of study data uncritically, or do they include methodological commentary along with their content review?

4. If authors have performed a meta-analysis or data pooling exercise, has their search for research studies been thorough? Have they

gone beyond simple computer searches of available databases to identify appropriate studies? Have they sought unpublished work as well as that published in non-English-language journals? In assembling their analysis, have they clearly identified criteria for study inclusion? Have data been extracted in a systematic and unbiased manner? Has the quality of studies under consideration been addressed? Has the possibility of publication bias been assessed?

This is a considerable list of queries. But by now most readers should be acquainted with the drill. Most of our problems in interpreting the literature can be traced to fundamental issues of selection and measurement bias. When these are held at bay, validity improves for any of the types of articles one encounters.

REFERENCES

1. Isner JM et al: Acute cardiac events temporally related to cocaine abuse. N Engl J Med 1986;315:1438.
2. Haller CA, Benowitz NL: Adverse cardiovascular and central nervous system events associated with dietary supplements containing ephedra alkaloids. N Engl J Med 2000;343(25):1833.
3. Raoult D et al: *Rickettsia africae*, a tick-borne pathogen in travelers to sub-Saharan Africa. N Engl J Med 2001;344(20):1504.
4. Warshaw GA et al: Functional disability in the hospitalized elderly. JAMA 1982;248:847.
5. Moses LE: The series of consecutive cases as a device for assessing outcomes of intervention. N Engl J Med 1984;311:705.
6. Bailar JC III et al: Studies without internal controls. N Engl J Med 1984;311:156.
7. Kappert U et al: Development of robotic enhanced endoscopic surgery for the treatment of coronary artery disease. Circulation 2001;104(12 suppl 1):I102.
8. Elul B et al: Can women in less-developed countries use a simplified medical abortion regimen? Lancet 2001;357(9266):1402.
9. Moertel CG et al: A clinical trial of amygdalin (Laetrile) in the treatment of human cancer. N Engl J Med 1982;306:201.
10. Relman AS: Closing the books on Laetrile. N Engl J Med 1982;306:236.
11. Aylett M et al: Stopping drug treatment of hypertension: Experience in 18 British general practices. Br J Gen Pract 1999;49(449):977.

12. Meier CR et al: HMG-CoA reductase inhibitors and the risk of fractures. JAMA 2000;283(24):3205.
13. van Staa TP et al: Use of statins and risk of fractures. JAMA 2001;285 (14):1850.
14. Meier CR et al: Statins and fracture risk. JAMA 2001;286(6):669.
15. Relman AS: Separating continuing medical education from pharmaceutical marketing. JAMA 2001;285(15):2009.
16. Adami S, Braga V, Gatti D: Association between bone mineral density and serum lipids in men. JAMA 2001;286(7):791.
17. Relman AS: How reliable are letters? N Engl J Med 1983;308:1219.
18. Sacks HS et al: Meta-analyses of randomized controlled trials. N Engl J Med 1987;316:450.
19. Haupt HA, Rovere GD: Anabolic steroids: A review of the literature. Am J Sports Med 1984;12:469.
20. Boule NG et al: Effects of exercise on glycemic control and body mass in type 2 diabetes mellitus: A meta-analysis of controlled clinical trials. JAMA 2001;286(10):1218.
21. Pettitti DB: *Meta-analysis, Decision Analysis, and Cost-Effectiveness Analysis: Methods for Quantitative Synthesis in Medicine*, 2nd ed. Oxford University Press, 2000.
22. Moher D et al: Assessing the quality of randomized controlled trials: An annotated bibliography of scales and checklists. Control Clin Trials 1995; 16(1):62.
23. Collaborative Group on Hormonal Factors in Breast Cancer. Breast cancer and hormone replacement therapy: Collaborative reanalysis of data from 51 epidemiological studies of 52,705 women with breast cancer and 108,411 women without breast cancer. Lancet 1997;350(9084):1047.

CHAPTER FOURTEEN

A
Final
Word

"When I use a word," Humpty Dumpty said in a rather
scornful tone, "it means just what I choose it to
mean—neither more nor less."
"The question is," said Alice, "whether you can make words
mean so many different things."
"The question is," said Humpty Dumpty, "which is to be
master—that's all."

LEWIS CARROLL, *THROUGH THE LOOKING GLASS*

As promised, we have worked our way through the major structure
of a medical article. We have sampled study designs and their strengths
and weaknesses, looked at the way data are collected and at some biases
that creep into that activity, and devoted considerable energy to critically
evaluating the way results are presented and analyzed. Along the way we
discovered many pitfalls that plague medical studies and journal articles.
We uncovered biases that occur because of selective recall, loss to follow-
up, and poor sampling techniques. We saw the untoward effects of
observer bias, the havoc wreaked by confounding factors, and the confusion created by misinterpretation of statistical significance.

We have honed our critical cutlery by learning something of random
allocation, stratification, control tables, and confidence intervals. In this

267

last chapter the accent will be on mobilizing the concepts of the previous pages into a final assessment of the value of an article. After all is said and done, is the information contained within the glossy pages worth retaining? We will also look at several resources to assist us in our critical considerations.

It has been mentioned before but is worth repeating that medical studies are rarely free from blemish. With our sharpened awareness, it is possible to find a tender spot in almost any article. The trick is to put skills to work in a constructive manner, balance the good points and the flaws, and decide upon a report's overall merit. Skills in critical analysis are easily abused. Without temperance, skepticism can degenerate into nihilism. That nets very little. On the other hand, as we pass from a thorough review of a study's methodology, through a careful evaluation of the collection of data and presentation of results, to the authors' discussion, we need to have confidence in our own abilities as reviewers. As authors put forth their interpretation and discuss the meaning of their work, we have every right to exercise our hard-earned judgment. If cynicism is a danger, so is self-effacement. Too often readers are willing to accept the views of medical writers and editors over their own reactions. Under intimidation by the experts, common sense is put aside. That is a mistake. The question, as Humpty Dumpty puts it to Alice, is "which is to be master?"

CLARITY

Most of us have had the unsettling experience of reading an article once and then a second time only to be left with the unhappy realization that we had no idea what the author was trying to say. Most often we take this to heart as a personal shortcoming: that a defect in our education or basic intellect is to blame for our failure to grasp the message. Rarely do we consider that it may be the writer's rather than the reader's deficiency. Medical articles are not always clearly written. Crichton has assailed medical writers for obfuscation, for camouflaging their communication in awkward prose and unnecessary complexity.[1] He says the effect of this bad writing is to make medical prose as dense, impressive, and forbidding as possible . . . the stance of authors seems designed to astound and mystify the reader with a dazzling display of knowledge and scientific acumen . . . what they (authors) are communicating is their profound *scientific-ness*, not whatever the title of their paper may be.[1]

Crichton's accusations that medical writers deliberately write obscurely to conceal thin papers and appear scientifically profound may smack of hyperbole, but there are seeds of truth. There is even some objective evidence to support his claims that medical minds can mistake bombast for wisdom. Researchers interested in the evaluations of medical students conducted several experiments assessing what has become known as the Doctor Fox effect.[2] In these studies, an actor was trained to lecture to medical students in a manner that would seduce them into feeling "satisfied that they had learned despite the presentation of irrelevant, conflicting, and meaningless content." The actor, dubbed "Dr. Fox," delivered his lectures with style, humor, and verve. They were, however, filled with "double talk, neologisms, non sequiturs, and contradictory statements." Students rating Dr. Fox gave his lectures highest marks in both style and content.

Impressed by the effects of the Dr. Fox experiment, Armstrong applied the principle to professional journals.[3] To test the hypothesis that "researchers who want to impress their colleagues . . . write less intelligible papers," he asked 20 business school faculty members to rate 10 management journals according to journal prestige. The readability of each journal was then assessed by applying a test of reading ease to sample articles. The test determined readability by sentence length and the number of syllables for each 100 words. Sure enough, there was a positive correlation between wordy, polysyllabic sentences and the estimated prestige. Because it might be argued that the content of the high-toned journals is more sophisticated and thus requires more elaborate prose, Armstrong added a second part to his experiment. He took concluding paragraphs from several articles and rewrote them, altering the readability but not the content. He sent these to another group of faculty members, asking them to rate the competence of the articles on the basis of the samples provided. Again, pedantry triumphed. Obscure writing tended to be rated higher in competence than simple, straightforward prose.

Although it may be unfair to generalize from management journals to medical writing, there is a message in this for medical readers. Clarity is the author's responsibility. If convoluted sentences and hazy verbiage obscure meaning, it is the writer's fault. Readers need to shake off the notion that their intellectual inadequacies are to blame when they have difficulty understanding a study. By the time most of us reach the stage where medical articles are appropriate reading, we are clever enough to understand them.

APOLOGIES, TENTATIVE CONCLUSIONS, SELF-CRITICISM, & THE LIKE

It is interesting to see how authors critique their own work in the discussion and conclusion sections of articles. Some authors are supremely certain of their results; others are overly modest. Blustering self-confidence invites close scrutiny when the author "doth protest too much." Results that are truly "obvious" or "self-evident" usually do not need the additional fanfare. Investigators' self-criticisms can range from empty apologies to insightful commentaries on the merits of the work. Some discussions contain so many modifying adjectives and qualifying phrases, the study swoons from dizzy indecision. "There may seem," "it might hopefully appear," "although evidence may be lacking," and "it may be generally considered to be" head a long list of qualifiers that weaken not only the writing style but the force of the message as well. Another kind of troublesome hedging occurs when, after laboring through the entire paper, we are told that the "results are only preliminary at this time," or that "the numbers studied may be too small to extract meaningful conclusions." Qualifications such as these are defended on the grounds that authors are trying not to overstate their case or make unsubstantiated claims. The intent is honest enough. Unfortunately, disclaimers that are tacked on to the final paragraphs of a piece offer readers no constructive alternatives for interpreting results. When authors quaver in their resolve, it shakes our confidence as well. We are left uncertain about the importance of the message. Do they really believe in their work? Is it useful news? How could it be improved or made meaningful?

On the other hand, genuine constructive criticism fosters confidence. It is reassuring when authors critically analyze their methods and interpretations. In a study reporting the "decreased risk of fractures of the hip and lower forearm with postmenopausal use of estrogens," Weiss et al head their discussion with a section entitled "Limitations of the Data."[4] They greet potential problems in this study head-on, describing possible biases and shortcomings in their work and assessing the effects of these upon interpretation.

In collecting information from cases and controls about estrogen use, systematic differences occurred. Women who had sustained fractures (cases) were interviewed on average 1 year after the fracture had occurred. However, they were asked to report estrogen use only until the time they sustained the broken bone. Controls, on the other hand, reported estrogen use until the time of interview. The authors worried that cases might have reported less estrogen usage because of the lapses of memory that occur with time rather than because of real differences in taking the medication. To attack this problem, they reanalyzed their data after removing the potential information bias. They dropped information about control subjects' use of estrogens for the year immediately prior to interview. Lower estrogen use among women with fractures was still demonstrated, supporting the beneficial effects of estrogens.

When we see references to "potential bias in our method" or accounts of "methods for controlling potential confounders," we can tell that authors share some of our critical concerns. Most authors are vested in their research hypothesis. They believe that estrogens reduce fractures and that treating high blood pressure reduces the risk of stroke. It is encouraging when they try alternative methods of analysis and still support their hypothesis.

CRITICAL ASSISTANCE

Consensus Statements

Medical journals are increasingly playing host to published consensus statements that advise us on a variety of topics from screening for dementia and treating scabies to guidelines for assessing the literature. Such recommendations come from groups of experts whose task it is to draw evidence together, evaluate it critically, and provide guidelines or recommendations on how to best proceed. Examples we have already encountered include the National Osteoporosis Foundation Working Group on Vertebral Fractures[5] and the CONSORT (Consolidated Standards for Reporting Trials) group that has published recommendations on reporting of clinical trials.[6] One of the more visible of the expert group efforts has been the National Institutes of Health (NIH) Consensus Development Program. The NIH began consensus development conferences in 1977. These conferences are convened to "evaluate available scientific information and resolve safety and efficacy issues related to biomedical technology."[7] The process involves 3-day meetings in which groups of expert investigators present data during open public session, questions and statements from conference attendees are discussed, and a panel of experts deliberates on the evidence and drafts an independent report. From the initial conference on breast cancer screening through recent conferences on management of menopause-related symptoms and chronic insomnia in adults, the series has attempted to provide evidence-based recommendations to the health professions. Statements are published in the *Journal of the American Medical Association* and as stand-alone reports. The high prestige of NIH and its ability to convene the highest level of scientific expertise to address each problem gives credibility to the proceedings. There are limitations as well. The consensus development process, it turns out, is not immune from nonscientific influences.

An important conference on breast cancer screening for women ages 40 through 49 was convened in January 1997. It was a timely conference given ongoing disputes among professional groups concerning the appropriate recommendations for mammography for women in this age group. Some were adamantly in favor of universal screening; others contended that evidence was insufficient to make such a recommendation. At the completion of the conference, after evidence had been presented, debate joined and the expert panel closeted, the recommendation came forward that the evidence was insufficient to support a recommendation for universal mammography screening for all women in their 40s.[7] Ten of the panelists endorsed this report, and 2 issued a minority statement endorsing routine screening.

The ink had scarcely dried on the report before a howl went up from Capitol Hill. Within days of the conference, the U.S. Senate voted 98 to 0 to endorse a nonbinding resolution that the National Cancer Advisory Board, which advises the director of the National Cancer Institute (part of NIH), consider recommending mammography for women in their 40s. From there a highly political sequence of events ultimately resulted in the National Cancer Advisory Board recommendation that the National Cancer Institute advise women in the 40–49-year age group who are at average risk of breast cancer to have screening mammograms every year or two. The expert panel's advice was overridden. The story is detailed in a journal commentary as a "clarion call for informed decision making,"[8] and suggests a type of bias we have not previously discussed.

Scoring Schemes & Rating Scales

The desire to improve the quality of published research has spawned numerous papers that focus on the process of critical review itself. No skin rashes are reported or remedies for back pain tested. Instead, these articles assess the quality of published research, and often, supply schemes for scoring methodological strengths and deficiencies.

An example is a report by investigators from the National Cancer Institute (NCI) that examines the quality of review articles published in the epidemiology literature.[9] In the last chapter, we decided that general reviews, which served the admirable purpose of summarizing knowledge on a particular topic, were susceptible to biases in the selection and interpretation of material included in the review. The NCI group tested that observation by scrutinizing the quality of 29 review articles published in 7 epidemiology journals. The authors rated each review using a published quality assessment guideline. Evaluated were such items as statement of search and selection methods, reporting of inclusion criteria, avoidance of bias and study selection, and reporting of criteria for assessing study validity. Results were not encouraging. Many of the reviews failed to meet quality expectations—a finding that was particularly troubling since authors of epidemiology studies should be particular sticklers for sound methodological practices.

A prominent feature of the quality assessment movement has been development and application of measurement tools such as the guideline just described. Clinical trials and meta-analyses have been particular targets for these assessments. The CONSORT group has already been mentioned for their guidelines to improve reporting randomized clinical trials.[6] The 22-item checklist they suggest is aimed specifically at improving reporting; however, there must of necessity be solid study design, execution, and analysis for high-quality reporting to occur. The checklist can guide not only authors who are reporting but also readers who wish to judge the quality of an article.

Checklists and rating scales have multiplied. This may be taken as a reassuring indication of the magnitude of the movement toward quality improvement, or as too much of a good thing. A review of the tools themselves revealed 25 scales and 9 checklists developed to assess the quality of randomized trials.[10] Most of these address common methodological concerns that we have discussed throughout the book: patient assignment, masking, follow-up, and statistical analysis, and so on. Considerable variation in the instruments is evident, however, in the number of items represented (3 through 34), scoring approaches, and methods of development. Authors of the review feared that despite the admirable goal of improving randomized controlled trials, the quality of many of the tools themselves was not high.[10]

Evidence supporting their concern surfaced in an exercise that compared performances of the scales. Juni and colleagues conducted a meta-analysis using 17 trials that evaluated 2 heparin preparations.[11] They then sorted these trials into bins according to their quality as rated by the 25 different instruments and repeated meta-analyses on the collection of high- and low-quality trials. They discovered wide variability and contradictory estimates of the benefits of the treatment depending on which of the quality scales was employed.

This is not to suggest that quality does not matter. It does mean, however, that proper assessment cannot be accomplished as automatically as checklists or scoring scales would imply. Limitations of the scales include the choice of items selected as quality indicators and the importance or weight that each is given. Not all strengths or flaws have equal importance. Nor are items in the scales always applicable. The trials that were included in the meta-analysis relating exercise and diabetes scored poorly on quality when rated by one of the standard scales.[12] However, the studies were docked for not properly blinding subjects and investigators— a task that is difficult to accomplish when the intervention requires going to the gym to lift weights 3 times a week.

Help from the Journals

With the awareness that informed readers require skills in critical analysis, several medical journals publish pieces that assist us in that task. Useful statistics primers such as "statistics for the non-statistician"[13] and "basic statistics for clinicians"[14] may be found in general-readership journals. Journals occasionally provide greater depth on particular topics that may puzzle us, such as confidence intervals or meta-analysis. These articles are targeted to health professional audiences and are generally "clinician friendly." The *Journal of the American Medical Association* (*JAMA*) has for some years offered an ongoing series called "Users' Guides to the Medical Literature." Authored by members of a consortium known as the Evidence-Based Working Group, these articles present thoughtful advice on how to use the medical literature to solve patient problems by assessing the validity and importance of evidence the articles present. The *Canadian Medical Association Journal* offers a series of "tips for learners of evidence-based medicine" that includes discussions of such familiar topics as relative risk and numbers needed to treat, confidence intervals, and measures of observer variability.[15] The *British Medical Journal* publishes a thick volume that concisely reviews the most recent evidence on the "effects of clinical interventions."[16] The tome has international authors and advisers and is updated every 6 months. Authors of the reviews are attuned to techniques of critical assessment, and reviews include estimates of the quality and strength of the evidence that underlies recommendations. Reviews are well referenced and a Web site is available.

Other groups have used the evidence-based approach to provide recommendations on screening and preventive health activities. There are both Canadian and American preventive health task forces that critically review research findings on topics from anemia to violence and make recommendations supporting or not supporting the activity. Each recommendation comes with an assessment of the quality of the evidence supporting their conclusions. The Canadian Task Force in particular publishes periodic updates in general medical journals and maintains an active Web site.

THE FINAL WORD

Regardless of how adamantly authors defend, support, deny, decry, declaim, apologize, or equivocate, we have a perfect right to disagree with their interpretation and offer our own. This disagreement over interpretation need not flow from problems with the paper's methods or analysis. It may simply be a matter of differing opinions over the importance of the findings reported.

Controversy over the recommendation on mammography screening for women between 40 and 49 years of age was not simply a disagreement over the evidence of screening efficacy. Summary data from 5 of the 8 clinical trials showed a small benefit (about 16%) to the screened group after 10 years of follow-up. However, when the relatively low incidence of breast cancer in younger women is factored in, the consensus panel calculated that "about 2500 women would have to be screened regularly to extend one life."[7] A U.S. Senate critic countered that "the panel appears to have lost sight of the human dimension of this question and gave undue weight to the cost of screening, rather than the benefits. The panel emphasized that 2500 women would have to be screened to save one life. But this one life represents someone's mother, wife, sister, or daughter."[17]

SUMMARY

We are back where we began—with a desktop full of journals, a desire to be knowledgeable, and a distressingly tiny aliquot of time. We have learned some analytic techniques and mastered our fears of inadequacy when confronting the experts. The task is formidable but not impossible. With a little planning, perseverance, and practice, we can make the medical literature not only palatable but downright digestible.

REFERENCES

1. Crichton M: Medical obfuscation: Structure and function. N Engl J Med 1975;293:1257.
2. Ware JE, Williams RG: The Dr. Fox effect: A study of lecturer effectiveness and ratings of instruction. J Med Educ 1975;50:149.
3. Armstrong JS: Unintelligible management research and academic prestige. Interfaces 1980;10:80.
4. Weiss NS et al: Decreased risk of fractures of the hip and lower forearm with postmenopausal use of estrogen. N Engl J Med 1980;303:1195.
5. National Osteoporosis Foundation Working Group on Vertebral Fractures. Assessing vertebral fractures. J Bone Miner Res 1995;10(4):518.
6. Moher D, Schulz KF, Altman D: The CONSORT statement: Revised recommendations for improving the quality of reports of parallel-group randomized trials. JAMA 2001;285(15):1987.
7. National Institutes of Health Consensus Development Conference Statement: Breast cancer screening for women ages 40–49, January 21–23, 1997. National Institutes of Health Consensus Developmental Panel. J Natl Cancer Inst Monogr 1997;22:vii.
8. Ernster VL: Mammography screening for women aged 40 through 49: A guidelines saga and a clarion call for informed decision making. Am J Public Health 1997;87(7):1103.
9. Breslow RA, Ross SA, Weed DL: Quality of reviews in epidemiology. Am J Public Health 1998;88(3):475.
10. Moher D et al: Assessing the quality of randomized controlled trials: An annotated bibliography of scales and checklists. Control Clin Trials 1995; 16(1):62.
11. Juni P et al: The hazards of scoring the quality of clinical trials for meta-analysis. JAMA 1999;282(11):1054.

12. Boule NG et al: Effects of exercise on glycemic control and body mass in type 2 diabetes mellitus: A meta-analysis of controlled clinical trials. JAMA 2001;286(10):1218.

13. Greenhalgh T: How to read a paper. Statistics for the non-statistician. I: Different types of data need different statistical tests. BMJ 1997; 315(7104): 364.

14. Guyatt G et al: Basic statistics for clinicians: 1. Hypothesis testing. CMAJ 1995;152(1):27.

15. Wyer PC et al: Tips for learning and teaching evidence-based medicine: Introduction to the series. CMAJ 2004;171:347

16. BMJ Publishing Group. *Clinical Evidence.* BMJ Publishing Group, 2005.

17. Gregorio DI: Refutation and conjecture around consensus breast cancer screening guidelines. J Public Health Manag Pract 1999;5(6):91.

Index

Page numbers followed by *f* or *t* denote figures or tables, respectively. Page numbers followed by *n* indicate footnotes.

Notes

Notes

Notes

Notes

Notes

Notes

Notes

Notes

Notes